CHANGE YOUR THINKING, CHANGE YOUR SHAPE

BEN WILSON

ISBN: 1463715560
ISBN-13: 9781463715564

CONTENTS

ACKNOWLEDGEMENTS

I would like to thank my mother and editor Vanessa Wilson. To Laura Young and Mille for reviewing the text and to all those who showed me support during the writing, including but not limited to James Cheeseman, Gareth Mason, Clive Wilson, Gina Wilson, Selma Prado and of course the cats for sitting here with me through the writing.

A special mention goes to my many clients who have listened to my stories of book writing and the many hundreds of people who I have met all over the world these last ten years. It is through their actions of getting into shape (or trying to) that I have been able to distinguish the different thinking patterns that underlie long term success.

DEDICATION

This book is dedicated to my Grandfather,
the late Aubrey Wilson.

INTRODUCTION

If you are reading this then you share my desire and that of many millions of other people - you want to look great, feel amazing and be proud of your body. It could be you want to lose a stone (14lbs /6.5kg) of body fat, have enough energy to keep up with your children or fit back into your clothes from a couple of years ago. Perhaps your goals focus more on developing a jaw dropping physique for the beach. Whatever your goals, I have written this book as an aid to help you achieve them.

Though the specifics may be different for each person, the theme of trying to improve your body is a goal which so many people strive to achieve but is only ever realised by a small percentage of people. If you look at the population today you will see that almost two thirds are classified as obese or overweight. Of the remaining third, only a small subset of people would be classified as being in amazing shape. The long term success rate of diets and weight loss attempts is horrendous. With so many people wanting to have a sensational body it raises the question as to why do so few people actually go on to achieve it?

Perhaps the best place to start looking for the answer to this question is through studying the behaviours of people who have achieved this cherished goal and are already in stunning shape. How did they succeed? What did they do differently to achieve their results? To create a high level of success in any field, it is important to understand what the high achievers did differently to their counterparts. This could apply equally in sports, acting, business or your body. This area has been extensively covered when it comes to financial success where you can find many books on the topic of how millionaires think differently to the rest of us. It is time to apply the same logic to how people in amazing shape think.

If thinking differently is the reason one person achieves a high level of success compared to another, then how do people of incredible shape think compared to the vast majority of people who are out of shape? If you can copy the thinking patterns of those that have enjoyed the greatest success in developing a sensational body then you too can create the same results

As a Personal Trainer, Nutritionist and Behavioural Change Coach I have benefitted from the opportunity of observing hundreds of clients over the years working both in a one on one capacity and group training environment. I have had people follow my advice and achieve their goals while others have spent lots of money to ignore everything I said. I have successfully helped clients lose lots of weight and maintain the results thereafter. I have also seen clients lose weight only to regain it all as they reverted back to old behaviours after we finished working together. Seeing these patterns time and again with my clients I decided to start studying the difference between those who were in shape and those who were not.

Working in gym environments for over 10 years I have had the opportunity to talk to literally thousands of people who ranged from body builders to housewives, professional athletes to business executives and fitness professionals to stroke victims. I have seen every type of body from jaw dropping six packs to 20 stone (280lbs / 127 kg) obese mothers. Meeting such people and many more in day to day life outside of the gym I was able to start to categorize the differences between how people in amazing shape think compared to their out of shape counterparts. I will be sharing that with you within this book.

I have written this book to help you create the results and changes within your body that you want to see. Whether this is losing 5 stone (70lbs /31Kg), dropping those last few pounds or developing the body of a fitness model it is the effectiveness of your mind set that will determine the probability of your success. If you adopt the thinking patterns of those with stunning bodies you will go on effortlessly to achieve your health and fitness goals.

If you want to achieve your health and fitness goals and achieve the body you always wanted you should use the following sequence:

1) Create a mindset so you can follow a nutrition and exercise regime.
2) Discover the right nutrition and exercise routine for you.
3) Follow this plan and adjust to allow for blocking factors as necessary.
4) Enjoy being in amazing shape.

This book is about taking that first step of creating the right mind set to allow results to happen. I am going to help you transform the way you look at food, exercise and health using the way successful people have done it as the formula for success. This book is as much about identifying and changing bad behaviours as it is about learning new ones. To change your behaviour you must first change the mindset that made you do the behaviours in the first place.

This book is arranged in four sections. The first section details the fundamentals of getting results and how to change both your mind and body. It outlines what influences success both physically and mentally. I discuss the true definition of being in amazing shape and how it goes way beyond what you can see on the outside. The issue of 'fake thin people' and how your mind works is also covered.

The second section highlights the many blocking beliefs that you hold around food, health and getting results. These beliefs are stopping you right now from going on to achieve success. They serve to keep us all out of shape. Break down these barriers and your mind will be free and open to think like someone who gets sensational results.

Section three details exactly how people in amazing shape think and how they act differently to the rest of the population. There are ten principles of thinking by which these people live their lives. The more of these principles and traits you develop within your personality, the better body you will possess both inside and out. This section also contains behavioural change exercises to help facilitate the cognitive changes you will be undergoing.

Section four contains your plan for moving forwards. It contains details on the strategies you will use to change your thinking and therefore change your shape. I set out the basic principles of the daily mind work out and show you what you should be doing within this daily mini mind workout to create dramatic changes within your body. Finally, there is a fifteen week results plan to accompany this.

This book is about change! The time for you to achieve your goals is now! This book works because it helps you change behaviours at a conscious, subconscious and emotional level which ultimately produces long lasting and dramatic body transformations.

Let's get started!

Ben Wilson

SECTION 1

THE FUNDAMENTALS OF CHANGING YOUR MIND AND BODY

This section introduces you to some of the fundamentals you need to know if you want to change your body and be one of the few people who get into amazing shape. When you have become aware of these fundamentals you will be able to more easily apply the things you will learn during the rest of this book.

WHAT IS BEING IN AMAZING SHAPE?

There are many different ideas and pictures of what being in sensational shape should look and be like. Differences exist between men and women, between age groups, cultures and individuals. The ideal body is often portrayed differently in the media than to what people really want to see in the real world. What do you picture when you imagine your dream body?

For some they just want to be thin, others want to be in shape but with curves while many want to be toned. Men often want that lean six pack look while some guys want an armour of muscle surrounding their frame. It is important you become clear on what you are trying to achieve.

At the very start of this book we need to clarify what I mean when I say someone is in 'Amazing Shape'. For me, being in great shape is more than just your external appearance. To be in truly great shape you must look great, but at the same time you must have the peace of mind to be able to enjoy it. This has to be accompanied by both strong health and good fitness.

The definition of being in great shape therefore has four elements; looking amazing, feeling amazing, possessing vibrant health and having a great level of fitness. Almost everyone focuses just on the external appearance (looking great) when it comes to picturing themselves and setting their goals. In fact, most people just picture themselves not looking the way they are, rather than focusing on creating what they actually want. The reality is that looking fantastic is the result of developing the other three areas.

Looking amazing	Feeling amazing
Vibrant health	Great fitness

Figure 1 – The four elements of being in amazing shape.

The way to look sensational is to possess vibrant health (nutrition and overcoming blocking factors) with good fitness (exercise) and to feel great (peace of mind, self acceptance, addiction /obsession free).

My definition of being in amazing shape is this:

"To have a body that makes you go WOW, which has great health, energy and fitness while also feeling happy about yourself and your body"

This target goes beyond your typical goal of losing a few pounds off your waist or having more energy. However that is exactly the point. Losing a few pounds off your waist is akin to the average person wanting to earn just 10% more next year. It is a minor improvement but goals wise it is not in the same ballpark as someone who is trying to make a million pounds within the next year. Your thinking patterns have to be completely different when you are shooting for the stars. Copy as many of the principles of people in amazing shape and your goal of losing a few pounds or increasing energy will be engulfed effortlessly on the way to greater things. Whatever your goals may be, look to copy the behaviours of people who are the very best in that field.

If you tune into your real desires you will hold a similar definition to what I am presenting. Everyone wants to look fantastic when they look in the mirror. While looking great is one thing you must feel as good as you look otherwise, what is the point?

You are going to struggle to feel good if you lack energy and suffer minor and/or major health complaints. We spend a lot of time suffering health issues and a lot of money on remedies for our headaches, coughs, colds, tooth aches etc. It is hard to feel ecstatic if these issues afflict your life. If your back hurts every morning or you have trouble walking without your knees creaking in pain, no matter how good you are looking you won't feel on top of the world. Looking great without feeling great is not living like someone who is truly in amazing shape.

Fitness is also an important component of being in great shape. Again this definition will vary for different people. For some it is being able to go for walks or picking up the grand children, while for others it is being able to run a marathon. Whatever your definition of fitness may be, it has to be included as an element of your health and fitness goals because it greatly contributes to both feeling and looking amazing.

Finally, and perhaps the most important element is your mind. It is vital you achieve peace of mind about your body. What is the point of looking like a movie star yet feeling like an ugly duckling? If you are going to be one of the very few people who do achieve their goals and possess a sensational body then what a complete waste to not actually enjoy it and instead spend your whole time telling yourself you are still overweight, need more muscle or that you need to change this bit or that.

Someone who is truly in amazing shape knows they are, this is not an arrogant statement but it is a truthful appraisal of the situation. By acknowledging your fantastic results you achieve peace of mind, confidence and an added enthusiasm to maintain results. You can never achieve peace of mind if you are telling yourself you are fat or ugly. If you are getting into good shape and edging closer to being in amazing shape you must acknowledge it. It is like a millionaire pretending he doesn't have any money in the bank. Why deny reality? Also, why wait for a specific goal to be achieved. Does the millionaire feel rich when he has £999 990 in the bank? Or should he wait until he has added that last 0.1% to his wealth to finally become a 'millionaire'? This is exactly what many do in regards to their bodies.

The enthusiasm to deny you look good is a significant contributor to people giving up their attempts to achieve the body they so crave. It is also the cause of one of the worst behaviours possible which is looking fantastic but not feeling it. When you have changed your mind set to match someone in amazing shape you will be able to truly embrace the situation so that when you do achieve your goal you will actually believe it and enjoy it.

As mentioned already I am teaching you how to create a mindset to create your dream body. This is not the same as just losing a few pounds and aiming for your 'goal' weight. Your goal weight is just the best of an average bunch. When aiming for the top, even if you "fail" you would have created a body in great shape and you would have made much more progress than someone who focuses upon attaining an average goal.

Your aim should be to shoot for the stars. To create a mind-body that is truly in amazing shape on all levels. It is irrelevant to your age, sex or financial status. The path to your dream body is open to everyone.

INFLUENCES ON BEING IN AMAZING SHAPE

Before identifying the main differences between those who are in shape versus those who are out of shape it is important to understand the basics of getting results. Being in amazing shape has two interrelated components. The actual process is a physical one yet it is your mind set that determines what physical actions you do or do not take. Thinking about losing weight will not get you into shape nor will thinking about eating a big cream cake make you any bigger. However, actually eating the right foods or the wrong ones will have an effect on your body. You can think about going to the gym all day long but the changes will not happen to your body until you physically do your exercise session.

Your thoughts form your behaviours and it is these actions which will determine what shape you are in. How do you think and act currently? Do you think about doing exercise and then get it done or does something always come up? Do you never think or even contemplate exercising? Do you think about eating chocolate? How do you react to this? Do you eat a big chocolate bar or avoid the temptation?

To be in amazing shape you will need to do a certain amount of the right behaviours for results while stopping enough of the wrong ones. For long term results you will have to incorporate these as lifelong behaviours and not short term changes. This is because only long term behaviours create long term results. The only way to ensure long term behaviours happen is to have those thinking patterns ingrained in your mind so that they are done naturally. Therefore working on your mindset needs more attention from you initially because the fact you are not in the shape you desire suggests you do not have the thinking patterns that produce results.

Mental influences on being in 'Amazing Shape'

The main mental influences can broadly be put into three categories. These combine to influence your physical actions. These are your emotions, beliefs and knowledge.

Emotions

Emotions are physical sensations within your body. They tell you how you feel about everything you encounter in life. This includes your food, exercise, your body and more. Your emotions are based on triggers, memories and beliefs created in the past.

Emotional connections are important because how you connect your emotions to certain actions will greatly increase the likelihood of a behaviour happening or not as the case may be. For example, if your connection to the local gym is one of excitement, enjoyment and happiness you are going to be exercising a lot more frequently than the person who has a connection of fear, embarrassment and pain to that same place. In terms of effortlessly getting in great shape you will need to feel a certain way about food, exercise and your body so that you naturally want to do the physical actions to be in great shape.

A second aspect to your emotions is your overall level of emotional stress. This is the total sum of all your emotions that surrounds your mind-body in any one moment. This represents the many thoughts, experiences and fears that you hold within your mind at any one time. This emotional stress is often at a subconscious level so you are not aware of it. When the total sum of your emotions becomes too great you will be forced to rely on addictive behaviours. This invariably involves food or drink and hence your excess emotions can prevent your long term success.

Beliefs

Your beliefs are made up from your past experiences, influences and acquired knowledge. Your beliefs act like a filter system to enable you to quickly process information and events you meet in life. The beliefs you hold will be totally natural to you and will seem like they are 100% right. The reality is our beliefs are simply opinions based on prior learning which may or may not be true.

Two people can have opposing and differing beliefs about exactly the same facts and information. The problem with our own beliefs is that once they are formed you will look for evidence in the world that supports your views. This is fine if your beliefs are such that they create the behaviours that will get you into amazing shape, but this is a disaster if they are not because you will be reinforcing the behaviour patterns that will keep you stuck where you are.

Knowledge

The final area of the mind is important in terms of getting into amazing shape because without the right knowledge and plan to follow you will struggle to achieve your goals whatever mind set you have.

Knowledge is most often thought of as coming from a textbook or some formal source of learning. This is one way in which we learn. However, the biggest way we learn in regards to health and fitness is not through text book style education but through our experiences in life, both what we see and what we feel personally. This is the area where we must pay most attention.

It is one of my goals in this book to educate you both formally (text book style minus the boredom, I hope) and through self experience. The latter is done by asking questions of yourself, observing other people, doing the exercises set out. If you follow my prompts you will experience the very things you need to learn to change your mind to get results.

Physical influences on being in 'Amazing Shape'

What you need to do to get into great shape depends on both your definition of what great shape is and of course where you are today. Regardless of your goal the most common factors are shown in figure 2.

To succeed you must eat the right foods and in the right amounts. This is elementary if you want to lose body fat or gain / develop muscle tone. You may be surprised about what a 'healthy food' is for your body because the traditional healthy living model has many inherent flaws as we shall discuss later in the book. As well as eating the right foods you will need to identify what foods are specifically dragging you down. This refers to food sensitivities which almost everyone has these days. In addition to nutrition, exercise is crucial to achieving an amazing look. Exercise takes different forms and can be a long way from the traditional view you may have down at your local gymnasium. What exercise you should do depends on your goals, likes/dislikes, biochemistry, injuries and facilities available. Either way, exercise has to be used to get into amazing shape.

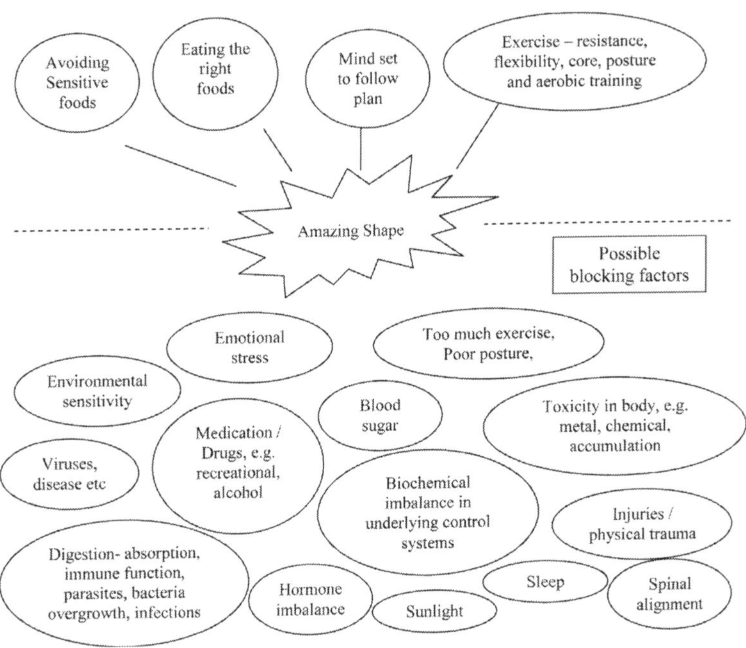

Figure 2 – Physical influences on being in amazing shape

Most people focus only on the issue of what foods to eat and what exercises to do when it comes to getting into shape. For a significant percentage of the population this alone is not enough to take you all the way towards your goals. This is because there are non nutritional reasons that affect your health and can prevent you achieving the body you want. These issues are called blocking factors.

When you are eating the right foods in the right amounts and following an exercise routine you would naturally expect to improve your health, lose weight and achieve the body you want. For many this is the case but for others this does not happen. Assuming the foods you are eating are actually right for your body then the only way to get results is to address and overcome the blocking factors in the way of your goal.

Most people simply give up when they run into blocking factors. The biggest hurdle for success is always your mind set which prevents you sticking to your plan in the first place and then taking it to the next level if you run into these hurdles.

Figure 2 outlines the many blocking factors that could prevent you from attaining the body you want. The diagram looks complicated because it outlines so many different possible factors upon success. These include blood sugar issues, metal toxicity, low vitamin D, posture issues etc. It is unlikely you will be affected by all of these problems but it is important for you to understand that even though you are following your plan correctly you may still need to go deeper into resolving these underlying blocks. There are different strategies that can be followed to overcome the different issues. How many of these and which ones apply to you will vary between individuals. The only way to see if they affect you is by following and adapting your nutrition and exercise plan. If you have tried all options yet not developed the body you want then you will know that these factors must be addressed.

People in amazing shape have solved the issue of what their body needs for results. The most important element for you to attain success and overcome possible blocking factors is your mind set. It is vital you do not quit before finding out what your body needs. This is what most people do and overcoming this issue is the focus of this book. For more details about these blocking factors I have provided some recommended reading in the further learning section.

HOW WE ARE THE SAME BUT VERY DIFFERENT

Almost everyone who has tried to get into shape has been overloaded with information and contradictions about all aspects of health. One of the main reasons there is so much conflicting / false advice in the world is because we are both the same as each other yet very different. This phenomenon is called Biochemical Individuality[1] and was coined by Dr Roger Williams. He reviewed thousands of medical studies. His work showed how we may be similar in many respects but we are also greatly different at the same time.

This can be seen in the way we all have eyes, nose, ears etc. yet no one looks the same as you. Two people will have different strengths and weakness both in their mental and physical abilities. The same thing applies to nutrition, do you notice how some people are always snacking and often feel hungry, yet others hardly ever feel hungry and can miss meals? Dr William's work proved conclusively how individuals can have vastly different nutritional needs from each other.

What this means in reality is because we are all very different there can be very few areas of advice that can be applied across the board to everyone. I will go into this in more detail in section three, but I wanted to explain early on why there is so much conflicting advice in terms of how to lose weight, gain muscle, healthy living and getting into amazing shape. It is because a certain strategy may work very well for some people, who then promote it as the best way forward based on their experience. This is fine, but be mindful that it just may not work for you. The key to success is discovering what works for you.

FAKE THIN PEOPLE

A consequence of how we are similar yet different at the same time is the issue of "Fake Thin People". They help in creating confusion in the advice on how to get into shape as well as sometimes being a negative influence upon you and your goals. A fake thin person is someone who is thin by luck rather than by effort. They give the appearance of being in great shape but this may have little to do with the methods they used to get there. There are four main types of fake thin people:

Type 1 – 'I can do anything and still be thin'

This type is most common with younger people. In your teens and early twenties you can often eat rubbish, drink, avoid exercise yet still be thin. I have met and worked with a few models and you would be surprised at how unhealthy most of them are. They are fake thin people relying on their bodies being resilient to putting on fat. Many of these fake thin people will eventually gain fat. However, some people will have low body fat for life however they act. This can be frustrating for you as you try to eat well yet will often have to see your friends eating all sorts of junk and somehow still stay in shape.

Type 2 – 'I look thin but I am actually overweight'

It may sound strange but if you measure people's body fat then you have a fairly equal measure of how 'good' someone looks without accounting for muscle tone. I have taken thousands of measurements on clients and have seen time and time again that you can have two people with the same body fat percentage but one person looks like they are in reasonable shape while the other person looks overweight.

People store body fat in different areas of their body. Therefore depending where you look or how you judge body fat someone can appear thinner than they actually are. For example some people store fat almost exclusively below their waist. This makes the upper body look thin while the lower body is larger. Depending on how you judge weight you can either be viewed as thin by looking above the hips or overweight by looking below. How you view people you meet depends upon your own views of being in shape and how you compare yourself to them. Often when looking at other people you will focus on their strong areas while ignoring their weaker areas. This means you may classify them as being thin because you looked at their better bits yet judge yourself as overweight because you focus on your worst bits.

Type 3 – 'I say I do nothing to be in shape but I put in plenty of effort'

This type of person is deceptive. They may portray that they do not follow a diet, limit foods or exercise yet they are looking great. At a party you may see them eating and drinking away like they have no cares in the world. However, if you examine them on closer inspection you will find they follow many of the principles you need to be in great shape. They are doing plenty of things that creates their look but they are either unaware that they do these things or they deny them for some reason. It could be it is so natural to them to not eat bread, avoid dairy, to train every morning before work that they never even think to mention it. Other people do not like to talk about what they do out of shyness or to avoid being challenged on their behaviours.

Type 4 – 'I am in shape but through a crazy obsession'

Getting into amazing shape does take some effort and the odd obsessive behaviour can come in handy. However there is a difference between a person who is doing it because he/she really wants to do that behaviour and someone who is doing it because they have to do it. It is the difference between wanting to go to the gym and feeling an almost obsessive compulsive behaviour to do so. The former brings peace of mind and enjoyment the latter brings resentment and conflict.

It is not that a bad thing for people to have achieved their great look this way, it is just there are easier ways to get there and you cannot copy their methods because you cannot choose to have an obsession. You cannot teach someone to create a fear of eating, a fear of fat, an hour a day minimum exercise obsession and why would you want to? These obsessive behaviors have not given the person peace of mind. They are in shape physically but not mentally.

Fake thin people and you

The point I want to make by mentioning fake thin people is that you should be careful who you listen to. It does not matter if someone is in shape through luck or effort, all that matters is how you react to these people and what they preach. Your path to possessing a sensational body both inside and out is a personal journey of discovery. Do not let the good appearance of others steer you from the correct path for your body. How to handle other people is covered later on as one of the ten principles of being in amazing shape.

I HAVE NO WILLPOWER!!

You may be thinking that there is no way you could do what it takes to get into shape because you simply do not have the willpower or the drive. This simply means you do not have enough of the beliefs that naturally produce the right behaviours for success. If you did you would not need to just rely on will power because you would naturally be doing what was needed without thinking about it. Willpower is only ever called upon when your beliefs (and therefore behaviours) are in conflict with what your conscious mind says you "should" be doing.

Your willpower helps you resist your cravings. Your long term success is how few cravings you are ever asked in the first place! Almost everyone has enough will power for results. Similarly, almost everyone does NOT have enough of the right subconscious belief patterns for long term results. Your success is not about how much will power you develop, it is about how many subconscious beliefs you create which automatically create the behaviours you need for results.

YOUR SUBCONSCIOUS BEHAVIOUR PATTERNS

Almost all your behaviours are done without actively thinking about it. This is vital for us to function as it saves us from having to think about how to breathe, walk or undertake everyday tasks. It becomes a problem with goal achievements when your automatic behavioural responses are not those that produce the results you want

Your mind immediately processes anything you encounter in life within a nanosecond by analysing the current situation versus your beliefs and then producing an emotion. The emotion you feel is designed to guide your behaviour in that situation, e.g. if feeling fear, proceed with caution.

The issue of willpower comes into play at this point. You can use your conscious thought (willpower) to overrule your emotional response. The larger the emotions the more will power needed to overpower them e.g. if you are craving chocolate you can "make" yourself resist it, the greater the craving the more will power you must have to resist.

In order to develop a body in amazing shape it is not about overcoming the emotion but rather cutting off the emotion at its source by changing the beliefs that created it in the first place.

The majority of people in society today possess a set of subconscious beliefs that limits their ability to get into shape. I refer to these as blocking beliefs and I discuss the major ones in section two. Conversely people in amazing shape possess a different set of subconscious beliefs which propels them onto success. These are discussed in section three.

To get in shape you must remove the blocking beliefs that are preventing your success and replace them with the ten principles of being in amazing shape. This will ensure your beliefs automatically create the behaviours that will change your body. Anyone can change their beliefs but you must become familiar with how to do this.

CHANGING YOUR SUBCONSCIOUS PATTERNS

For you to develop the thinking patterns of someone in amazing shape you can use the following five stages to changing your subconscious programming. These are awareness, questioning, intention, planning alternative strategies and emotional management.

Awareness – You must become aware of how you act and what you believe. You can then become aware of more productive strategies that are available to you. This whole book acts as a task in awareness. Bringing your attention to faulty beliefs and behaviours you possess currently and more productive strategies other people hold.

Questioning – You should begin to question gently why you have your beliefs and why you do not have more productive beliefs.

Intention – You need to decide what new behaviours you want to create and what beliefs would underpin these.

Organised planning – You will need to plan consciously and work out how to change many of your old behaviours into new more productive behaviours. This may take some thinking, planning and testing of what works for you.

Emotional management – The final and perhaps most important element is to change the emotions about your old behaviours and desired new ones so that you naturally want to do the right behaviours. This desire must occur at an emotional level for long term results. This is the ultimate goal of subconscious behavioural change process.

There are various strategies and methods that can be used within each of the five stages. These can include techniques to break down emotions, affirmations or simply writing down your thoughts around an issue. I will be introducing you to many of these during the rest of this book.

FEELING EMOTIONAL

Your emotions are crucial to success because they determine how you will act in the majority of situations. We allow our emotions to guide us in how to act and this is equally as likely to draw us into eating some cake as it is to take us down the gym. To counter this type of emotional influence you must focus on changing the beliefs that create this emotion in the first place as discussed already.

A second element to emotions is the level of emotional stress you are experiencing. Most people confuse emotional stress with how busy they are at the moment or if they are going through a tough time. However, the sum of your emotions is much more than this. It comes from many more angles than just what is going on in your life at the moment.

Your mind-body has a certain level of emotional stress that it can cope with naturally. When emotions run above that level you will need to rely on addictive behaviours. This is where most people run into problems. The addictive behaviour they rely on when emotions run high is usually eating the very foods that prevent you getting results. This interplay can be seen in figure 3.

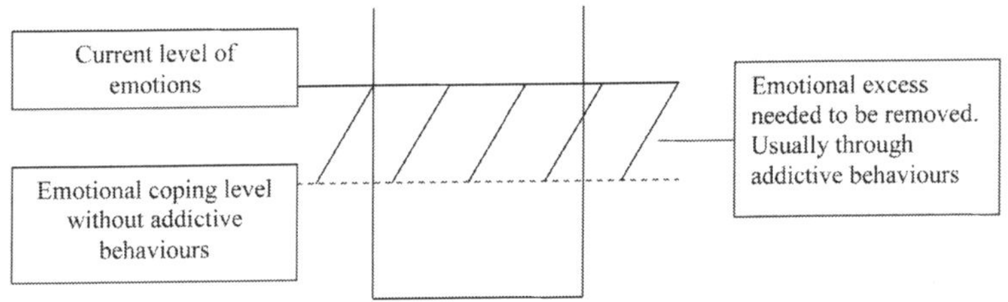

Figure 3 – Levels of emotion and coping ability

To prevent your emotions sabotaging your goals of getting into shape you need to reduce the amounts you are experiencing while simultaneously improving the coping strategies you use. To do this you must be aware of your emotional stress and the influence this has upon you.

Your Emotional Stress

Your total level of emotional stress is made up from emotions generated from your past, present and future. This is shown in figure 4. The less negative emotions you experience the easier it is to stick to your nutrition and exercise routine. Therefore this is a crucial area to control in order to attain success. People in amazing shape have found a way to handle their emotions in a more productive way to their out of shape counterparts.

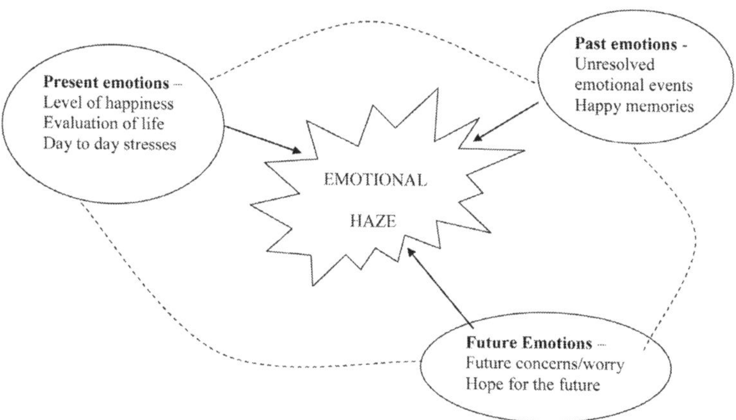

Figure 4 – Influences on your emotional stress

As you can see, the level of emotions you experience stems from many different sources. These emotions are often buried within your subconscious so you are not really aware of them having a negative effect upon your mind-body. The more you understand the possible contributions the more effective you can become in reducing your emotions and therefore increase adherence to your regime.

Past events

Your past contributes to your emotional stress in terms of unresolved emotional events. An unresolved event is any moment from your life which if you think about today still evokes negative emotions. The average person has hundreds of these from small things such as being annoyed at your friend for not paying you back the £20 he owed you, to guilt, sadness or regret about major things that have happened within your life. This includes emotions about events and decisions you have / haven't made in your life.

Present day emotions

This refers in part to the day to day stresses and demands put upon you. It includes deadlines in work, getting the kids to school, taking the dog to the vet, moving house or any other activity that takes up your time and focus. These can be good or bad events, stressful or fun. It is the things you face in your daily life.

Another aspect of your present day emotions is your current evaluation of life. This is the relationship of your expectations versus evaluation within the different areas of your life. Your evaluations can contribute emotions of stress into your mind-body (figure 5).

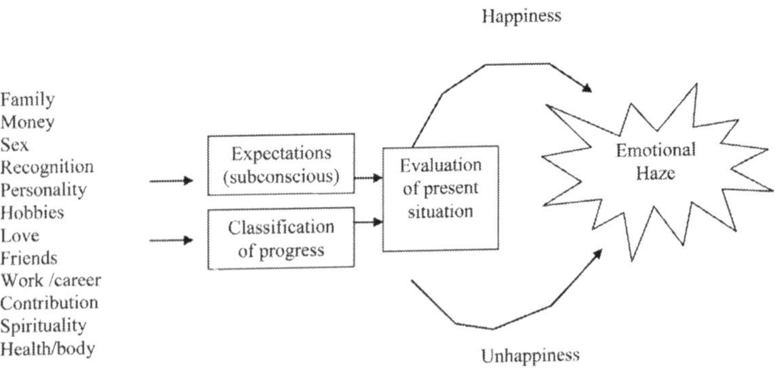

Figure 5 – Evaluations of life and their contribution to your emotional stress

The key to whether you experience stress or positive emotions from your current evaluation is based upon your expectations. Without classification and expectations you cannot experience emotions about an issue. If you are a size 10 dress size it can only have meaning depending on what your expectations are. If you expect to be a size 6 then you can feel very unhappy about being a size 10. If you had not expected to lose weight and return to a size 10, you could feel very proud and happy. It is the same dress size but only the evaluation and classification that has changed.

In other areas of your life you will have many goals and expectations about what you should achieve. This could be the amount of money you want to make, your relationship to your family, progression in your career, sex and fulfilment of sexual desires amongst many other possibilities. These thoughts are often hidden in the subconscious and therefore you do not necessarily spot them.

They can often increase in importance on landmark birthdays. Often people get depressed when they reach 30, 40, or 50 years old because they evaluate where they are in life versus their prior expectations of where they thought they would be and this often produces a negative feeling. Any negative feelings produced will add to your emotional stress.

Future concerns

The final area of contribution to your emotional stress comes in the form of thoughts about the future. As human beings we spend a lot of time worrying about future events. As the saying goes "I have had many worries in my life, most of which never came true"

There are two main types of future concerns, the short term day to day worries and long term thoughts about life/death/spirituality etc. People do not like uncertainty and hence future concerns are a great source of emotional discomfort. Most of us are aware of our worries about the day to day events that are happening, e.g. getting to work on time, giving a presentation or not having enough money to pay the rent.

Long term future concerns are often more subtle. They often centre on answering questions about life and your future. These are the type of questions which do not have definitive answers. Whether you consciously think about it or not we all have thoughts regarding death, what happens after death and the meaning of life. The problem with these types of questions is that there is no way of knowing the answers. This is not good for our peace of mind as we thrive on understanding. This lack of knowledge can be a significant source of negative emotions to some people.

Handling your emotional stress

If you want to get into amazing shape then you will need to address your emotions in one way or another. Some people will need to focus on this area more than others. The key to success is how you reduce the negative emotions experienced. To do this there are various techniques that can be used. This includes Emotional Freedom Technique (EFT), Thought Field therapy (TFT), Neuro-Linguistic Programming (NLP), Cognitive Behaviour therapy (CBT), Psych-K and many therapist based techniques amongst others. Another route is to look into the nature of stress and thought as covered by "The Three Principles". We will discuss some of these further in the book and more information on all these can be found in the further learning section. Another way to counter negative emotions is simply by becoming happier.

HAPPINESS

The natural counter to negative emotions is feeling happy. It is an important area when it comes to being in amazing shape because the way you handle any unhappiness in your life can prevent you achieving the body you want. Most people resort to eating the very foods that prevent success when they are unhappy. To counter this you should therefore look to increase ways of being happy. The term happiness is a broad term which describes the general feeling you get when you feel good. If you dig a little deeper you can identify four types of happiness. These are pleasure, satisfaction, fulfilment and enlightenment.

Pleasure – This is a short term good feeling. Pleasurable activities range from a day out at the beach to reading a book. It can be anything from going to the cinema, relaxing with friends, listening to music, sex, eating, hobbies and many more activities. They also include more detrimental behaviours to your health such as eating a cake, smoking a cigarette or drinking a glass of wine. Pleasure is the shortest lived of the happiness emotions, it is the easiest to obtain and affects us the least deeply.

Satisfaction – This is the feeling you get from the accomplishment of a task. The feeling comes after the event and can occur even if the task was not enjoyable at the time. You can feel satisfied from playing a good game of tennis, talking to your friend, cleaning the house or painting the garden fence. Satisfaction lasts longer than the feelings of pleasure.

Fulfilment - This feeling comes from the 'success' we have achieved within specific areas of our lives. This could be the feeling of fulfilment at having become manager in your job or having three wonderful kids. This feeling does not need real world "success" to be experienced. You can short cut to this feeling by following your inspiration. The more inspired you feel in your life the more fulfilled you will feel. Most people today have forgotten what inspires them and instead do the tasks they feel "should" give them inspiration.

Enlightenment – This is where love, joy and acceptance are flowing within the body. It is when you have reached true fulfilment in all areas of your life. It is living in the now. Enlightenment also brings peace of mind on both the past and the future. This state is referenced in various religions. The short cut to this feeling is through giving out unconditional love (giving love without that long list of things that must happen in return for it). This is the longest lasting and deepest level of happiness.

Increasing happiness

While this may all sound a bit spiritual and airy fairy for some people, as humans, we have an innate desire to achieve and experience happiness. We all strive subconsciously to achieve enlightenment (experience unconditional love). If we cannot achieve this we will try to experience fulfilment (inspiration). When this fails we will look to satisfaction and pleasure to feel good. The most common way to add pleasure to our lives is through food and this becomes a problem because we rarely choose the foods that help our body. This is why it is important to try to increase your levels of happiness as much as possible within your life and thus avoid relying on food to feel happy.

In our favour is that happiness is our natural default state. We do not need to do anything specific to feel happy but more we need to stop doing the things that distracts us from our happiness. A baby is always happy until something takes this feeling away temporarily (hunger, temperature, needs changing etc). Once resolved the baby returns to happiness. We as adults are the same. Left to our own devices we will feel happy but we are distracted through our thinking, physical pains/aches, stresses of life etc. Through engaging the different aspects of happiness described above we able to bypass these distractions from our happiness.

SECTION 2

BELIEFS THAT BLOCK SUCCESS

You will recall that your beliefs are the thoughts and opinions you have about the world around you. They control how you behave in the vast majority of situations. There is no such thing as a right or wrong belief but rather that certain beliefs will help you attain a goal while others will block your progress.

When it comes to getting into shape there are certain beliefs that will prevent you achieving success. For you to improve your results you will need to remove these from your mind set. I have outlined the major blocking beliefs within this section. People who are out of shape believe these more strongly than those who are in shape. As a result they are destined not to have the body they desire.

Many of these blocking beliefs are formed during childhood alongside the majority of our other beliefs about life. However, much of the beliefs relevant to achieving a body in great shape are learnt in adulthood. The main source of this learning comes from the media and general customs of our culture.

If you are reading this book and are not currently in the shape you would like to be then you can almost take it as given that you are holding many of the blocking beliefs that are preventing you getting the body you want. To prepare yourself for learning and absorbing the ten principles of how people in amazing shape think you will need to clear your mind by breaking down your blocking beliefs. This section is designed to make you aware of these beliefs so you can drop them from your mindset.

The following beliefs are in no specific order but they are all common blocking beliefs that society in general holds. The less you have of these, the easier it will be to get the body you want.

BLOCKING BELIEF - FOOD MAKES ME HAPPY

Eating food to make you happy can be a big block on achieving your goals. Everyone will feel disappointed, sad, annoyed, angry, guilty, regretful and jealous among other emotions at some point during their life and these feelings will make you feel temporarily unhappy. If your response is always to grab food when you experience these situations then your body will suffer.

When I say "food" I mean the typical foods people grab when they feel down. If we all ate celery when stressed this belief would not be an issue. However that is rarely the case. Most people instead rely on "comfort foods" which invariably have disastrous effects on the body.

It is not possible to go through life without experiencing negative feelings. The most effective method if you want to be in amazing shape is to understand the brain washing you have had about food making you happy and to use alternative strategies other than eating when you are feeling down.

Food can generate a genuine pleasure feeling or a false pleasure. Figure 6 shows the different ways of using food for happiness in relation to the four types of happiness scale.

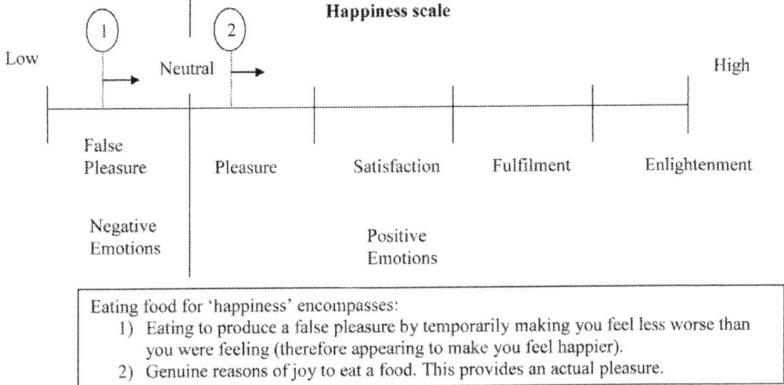

Figure 6 – Food, false pleasure and the happiness scale

Eating food for happiness gives either a low level of pleasure e.g. that food tastes nice, or it provide a false pleasure, e.g. makes you feel not quite as bad as you were feeling previously. The pleasure provided from food is very short lived. Therefore, if you rely solely on it as your pleasure source (especially false pleasure) you will return to it frequently and often (because you still feel unhappy).

Believing food makes you happy often creates a catch 22 situation. You feel upset because you are out of shape and thus eat foods to feel better which then makes you further out of shape and more upset.

Put another way your favourite food which you think makes you happy or is pleasurable is in fact a major contributor to your lack of fulfilment and dissatisfaction in life. The very food you think is your friend is the actual cause of you being out of shape. It perpetuates your low self confidence, poor energy and health problems. The question is how long will you continue to let this food bring you down and away from the real person inside? The person who looks and feels great, the person who believes in themself and is truly happy......the true you!

It is hard to believe food makes you in happy in the face of such evidence. The problem is whether you view the food on a short term scale (during and a few moments after eating) or in the longer view of consumption (from 20-30 minutes after eating onwards). If using the latter then there is no way you can hold the belief that food makes you happy. As both views are valid it is important to not only focus on the short term benefits without consideration of the longer time period. Food may taste nice and provide a pleasure but it does not make you happy. It is important to understand this difference.

Many people appreciate this logically, but struggle to appreciate it emotionally. Some people hold firm in their belief that food does make you happy. The more you believe that food makes you happy the more out of shape you are destined to be.

Finding pleasurable activities in your live is easy. Many tasks can be pleasurable, such as going for a walk, spending time with your children, playing with the dog, watching your favourite TV show, sex, hobbies, exercise and many more activities too numerous mention here. When you can see that food is just one of many pleasurable activities and possible options it should allow you to explore other avenues of happiness. Using food for happiness as one of many options will still allow results to happen, using food as your only option for happiness will not.

Do you know which pleasurable activities are the ones you enjoy the most? It is the ones that engage the higher levels of happiness. It is the activities that not only provide immediate pleasure but also provide satisfaction and fulfilment (inspiration). These are the tasks that truly give joy. However, despite this, you may keep on returning to eating for your happiness. This is often caused by emotional anchors.

Anchors

An anchor is a physical trigger that evokes an emotional reaction from the mind-body. It is the role of emotional anchors that makes many people eat for happiness even if they know that food does not make them happy. The role of anchors is very powerful to our mind and greatly influences behaviour patterns.

You may be familiar with anchors from the studies by Russian physiologist Ivan Pavlov and his dogs. In the experiment he would ring a bell each time he gave the dogs their food, before too long he would ring the bell (physical stimulus) and it immediately produced the emotions of eating within the dogs (anticipation of food, excitement, salivation etc) regardless of whether there was any food in the room or not.

As humans we are exactly the same. Different triggers will evoke emotions from the past. You will experience this when you hear a song that reminds you of a good time, the song makes you feel good now. Alternatively, a "sad" song may remind you of a negative experience and upset you. A person's mannerisms may remind you of your parents or a good friend and this will cause you to react in a certain way. Anchors produce immediate emotional responses direct from the subconscious.

Almost everyone has emotional anchors connected to food. When a certain food is eaten it reminds you of a time from the past. I always associate Christmas with Quality Street chocolates and trifle. Christmas is the best time of the year for me. It is always fascinating to see how the cravings for these foods will appear at other times during the year and especially if there is a lot of stress in my life.

It is important to remind yourself that your brain is very clever and every strategy you currently undertake is simply the best strategy your mind has come up with using your current knowledge and circumstances. Every behaviour you do serves an exact purpose. Do not criticize yourself for eating chocolate when you are upset, it is just what your brain has come up with as the best coping strategy it could find so far. The problem is that your best strategy may be disastrous upon your body. It may also be fairly ineffective at achieving the desired emotional outcome your mind wants.

Anchors can cause mischief because the feelings they induce will be ones of happiness and good times. This will give the illusion that the food is making you happy. In reality it is reminding you of good times from before. It is no different to playing your favourite song from your youth or reminiscing with your friends about good times that you had in the past.

This is where you must understand the food is not the provider of happiness but it is the memory of the previous event or time period in your life. Many people eat foods to remind them of childhood, a time where we remember what life was like without the stress, worry and responsibility of adulthood. There is nothing wrong with remembering good times from the past except when using food to do so it will have a negative impact on your body.

Anchors are further developed if you reach for your favourite food when you are feeling happy from other events in life. It will connect happiness to eating that food. The same is true if you grab your favourite food whenever you are really hungry or low on energy. It will perk you up (as almost any food would do in that situation) and thus further reinforces the good feelings provided from your 'happy' foods.

Setting up your own anchor

As food is such a strong anchor for happiness, an effective way forward is to fight fire with fire by developing your own anchor that can induce good feelings or memories without involving food. This way you can use emotions to combat the craving for food. A process for setting up an anchor is outlined below. Follow this example to create an anchor for happiness. This same pattern can be used to create other anchors, e.g. relaxation:

- Choose a spot on the body, e.g. hold together your left thumb and first finger.
- Now sit back and make yourself comfortable. Begin gently holding the anchor point (e.g. thumb and first finger) and close your eyes.
- Take two minutes to think back to a time where you experienced high levels of happiness. It can be helpful to play some music and if possible use scents and aromas that remind you of these happy feelings / times of your life.
- Continue to hold the thumb and first finger of the left hand together and now take another two minutes to think about how happy you will feel in times to come. Let your mind vividly imagine it and feel these great feelings of happiness that will be happening to

you in the future. Again include music and scents if possible to further enhance the imagery.

- Anchors can be quick to form but it usually takes practice to create a strong anchor that is of any real use to you. Repeat this exercise several times. The more intense the emotions you experience during the past and future imagery the more effective your anchor will be.
- Once established you can re touch the anchor point to make you feel happy by reminding yourself of these feelings.

When an anchor is set up and working effectively you can simply touch and rub the anchor point whenever you need a positive emotional reminder. This will reduce and ideally replace the desire to eat a food to evoke that same memory. There are also natural anchors you can make use of to achieve this objective, things like listening to music, looking at old photos, doing a hobby, visiting old haunts. Well developed anchors can fit nicely in the overall process of creating a mindset destined to get you in amazing shape. Anchors are not the total solution but a handy tool to use alongside other techniques.

The goal of removing the belief that food makes you happy is to allow you to open yourself up to the other possible pleasurable activities you can do in life. Dropping this belief does not mean that you will never eat junk food ever again, it allows you the option of not having to eat it and thus the food becomes just one strategy amongst many others.

BLOCKING BELIEF – IT IS EXCITING TO EAT JUNK FOOD

People in poor shape will often comment how strict or boring a healthy lifestyle may be and that they find it exciting to eat other less healthy options. While I can understand how they have formed their point of view I also know they are looking at the picture the wrong way round.

When reviewing the success and thrills over the last year you will find that eating that bit of cake September 28th, 11.37am will not necessarily rank up there in the terms of your most exhilarating moments. Eating food for excitement is a terrible way to make up for a lack of excitement in other areas of your life.

Most people find they eat food in search of excitement during the everyday tasks of work, home life, waiting to pick up the kids from school and so forth. When people eat for excitement in these situations it is to suppress the negative feelings of boredom rather than for the joy the food brings. Eating to mask a feeling is not the same as eating to experience a feeling.

If you are eating to mask an emotion, it is characterised by consuming very similar foods time in time out. After 100 bits of cake you would have thought the true excitement would have worn off. Would you watch the same TV episode a 100 times? Unfortunately, the excitement does not necessarily wear off because each time you eat the cake you are masking the underlying emotion and thus providing temporary relief, which in turn gives a false feeling of excitement. Sometimes you eat simply because it is something to do. This is another form of food being used for excitement.

Eating to experience a feeling (as opposed to deadening an emotion) is an action borne out of excitement. It relates to trying new foods, restaurants and cooking techniques. The goal is to experience the tastes of food. When eating this way variety becomes the key. You want to try different techniques, foods and tastes. This style of eating provides you with an actual pleasure by trying the new foods and the satisfaction from making it etc. This style of eating forms the basis of the many thousands of cook books and cooking shows on TV. When this is combined with the social fun of dinner parties and social events you can see how the term eating for excitement could be coined.

If you are going to claim that eating is exciting then you must also acknowledge the host of boring aspects it brings too. These include the constant feelings of low energy, digestive problems, food cravings, headaches, being out of shape and having poor mental alertness. How much worry, angst and concern does this cause you? Aren't you bored of looking in the mirror and thinking you are overweight? Tired of feeling awful and having low energy? Every time you eat in search of excitement to brighten up a dull moment you have to think would your life be more exciting already if you didn't have those ongoing boring problems? Each time you use food as a prop because you are bored you are actually creating a vicious circle in your life by continuing those tiresome health complaints that keep dragging you down.

People often comment it is boring to eat the same healthy foods all the time yet most people eat just a handful of different foods as part their "non healthy diet". The food plans I provide to clients have over 370 different foods listed yet most people complain because their two favourite foods are eliminated from the plan without even looking at the other 368. When you have removed your attachments to using foods for false pleasure you can open up your mind to trying the hundreds of different foods out there. When you stop using food for excitement you can start to follow a healthy diet without being bored with it.

To counteract using food for excitement you need to look at increasing the overall levels of excitement in your life. In addition to this you must also create alternative strategies and behaviours to do when bored to replace the times you would have just eaten food. When combining this with the expanding list of foods you consume you will be able to break this blocking belief.

BLOCKING BELIEF – FOOD HELPS YOU TO RELAX

Many people use junk foods to help them relax at the end of the day, on the weekend or perhaps in the midst of a stressful day. It is no surprise we resort to food in an attempt to relax our mind-body because we are living in a world of more stress and less peace of mind than ever before. The only problem with using food to relax you is that it has very limited benefits in terms of relaxation and of course ruins your body in the process!

What is your picture of complete relaxation? Take a moment to picture it.

What did you think of? Maybe you thought of being on holiday on a beach, away from it all, maybe you pictured yourself at home with some music playing or walking in the country.

Whatever scene you pictured, there is normally a common theme running through images of complete relaxation. These are that are you are away from life's stresses, your own thoughts about life seem different, you have less worries, you are away from work, the daily hustle and bustle, the crying kids, the household chores etc. All that daily noise and stress is suddenly silent and you can just relax. This is what relaxation means, getting away from the current stresses in your life. It is about quietening the mind, being free from worry and at peace. This is why we love holidays. We go away and it takes our mind off the problems in our life for a short while.

It is for a similar reason most people use food as a diversion for their mind. When eating your thoughts become focused on the task at hand and this mental diversion will very temporarily take you away from your problems. This is further enhanced from the food anchoring into memories and emotional states which also divert your mind. As is always the case with food the temporary distraction soon wears off, sometimes in no more than a few minutes and then you are back to face the stresses of life.

A problem with using food for relaxation is the catch 22 situation it creates. Any addiction creates additional stress to the mind-body in the times that you are not doing the addictive behaviour. For example, a long term smoker often smokes because he thinks it 'relaxes' him. When a smoker is not physically smoking a cigarette they are experiencing additional anxiety caused from not doing the addictive behaviour. Therefore anytime he is not smoking he is experiencing stress. This is independent of what is happening in his life. Therefore the smoker will smoke whether he is happy, sad, stressed or relaxed, because he must remove the stress of not smoking.

The same can happen with food in that the only time you are not craving the food source, e.g. sugar, chocolate, cake etc, is when you are eating it. This is because it is the only time you do not experience the anxiety of "not doing" this activity. This is added on top of all the other stresses you have from life which may make you want to eat to get away!

At some point you have learnt to use these strategies to try and relax. Where one person drinks each night another person goes to the gym. Some people read while others eat cake. There are no rights or wrongs to this. But let's make it clear, certain strategies will totally destroy your efforts of losing fat and being in great shape. They will sentence you to a life of feeling bad and unhappy about how you look in the mirror. The wrong relaxation strategies can mean you have to continue being overweight and out of shape. This will ultimately create an even greater stress which you will need to relax from.

Food does not relax you! If you look at the big picture, using foods to relax simply increases the amount of stress in your life by subsequently making you less able to handle events emotionally (a side effect of eating poorly) and by making you overweight, which further creates more stress in your life!

Food gives the impression it relaxes you by masking the stresses in your mind for a very short period. This is not relaxation. This is suffering slightly less stress than before. True relaxation comes from doing something to engage the mind in alternative thoughts. True relaxation comes from breaking down the emotions and worries affecting you. It is a misconception that if you want to de-stress then you can just sit down and do nothing. The brain does not work like that. If you do not believe me try this experiment. When you are on your own turn off everything that can possibly disturb you e.g. phone, TV, children, pets etc and then simply sit there in a chair and do nothing. Do not fall asleep but sit there awake. Then listen to your mind. It will continually be producing thoughts, listen to them. Most people find this uncomfortable, they are alone with their thoughts and they are shouting at you!

When you are eating to relax you are trying to mask these thoughts. It is no different to turning on the TV. What both these techniques try to do is distract your mind from thinking by diverting attention. The problem is these methods are so weak at distracting your mind it is barely worth doing. Once the food has been consumed the thoughts will generally begin to resurface. Then what do you do? Eat to relax once more? If you have used this behaviour for a while that is exactly what you will do.

True relaxation comes from ensuring the mind is quiet. This is done by engaging the mind in another activity (as opposed to sitting there passively trying to mask your thoughts) or through actively trying to reduce the emotion. Meditation is also a powerful way to relax the mind. You do not need to be a monk sitting in a cold dark room. The basic principle of meditation is to focus on your breathing and then to use the mind to direct your thoughts. In this sense exercise, dancing, singing and playing sports /games are all forms of meditation along with the more tradition style techniques. The safest and surest method for relaxation is to spend as much time doing activities that you find truly inspiring and exhilarating. This will engage your mind, fill you with excitement and reduce your levels of emotions.

BLOCKING BELIEF - ALCOHOL

The beliefs about alcohol follow along similar lines as believing that food relaxes you or makes you happy. There is a difference though, alcohol significantly changes your mental outlook (physiologically) and alters your experience of life. It is a drug, society's second biggest drug of choice behind food.

There is a difference between drinkers and how they behave around alcohol. Some have a glass once in a while, others drink daily, while some follow the binge drinking route. If alcohol is a block towards your goals then it needs to be addressed. In general alcohol becomes a major problem for most people's goals when you drink every day or you are caught up in the binge drinking lifestyle / culture. If you have an occasional glass of wine once or twice a week it is unlikely to impede your goals in most circumstances.

People drink for five main reasons. Some drink because they lack confidence to act a certain way sober while others because they are trying to forget about life e.g. suppress their emotional stress. Many individuals have simply developed the belief it is fun, relaxing or makes them happy. Other people drink because of nutritionally based cravings (though most are unaware this is the reason) while a proportion of drinkers do it for the social inclusion in a group or sense of community it provides.

Drinking to gain confidence is a cry for help from your mind and a problem that can be resolved normally with just a few simple self development techniques. If you are drinking for confidence then you have three options really, drink for the rest of your life whenever faced with this situation, avoid this situation for life or develop yourself to avoid needing to drink in that situation. The easy way out is to resort to drink. The difficult yet infinitely more fulfilling solution is to develop yourself so you can handle the situation. Whether it is to speak to someone you find attractive, to dance, to have sex or be able to tell someone how you feel. The ability to deal with these situations sober is an amazing experience. It takes some effort, some growth to be able to change from the person who needs alcohol to the person who doesn't but it is worth the effort. This process may not happen overnight but once you have started you are on the path to succeed.

If you drink to avoid a problem or because of the current state of your life, you are making life much more difficult for yourself. Drinking does not solve the problem as I am sure you are aware, in fact it makes it worse. Drinking alters your mental outlook causing a more depressive forecast on the problems at hand. Disrupting the body's biochemical balance (via food or drink) makes you less apt at handling events emotionally or logically. The problem you are trying to forget is of course still there however much you drink it out of the foreground.

If you are trying to forget about life, an event, or generally reduce your emotional stress by masking it with alcohol then listen to the call for support from your mind-body. When drinking because of excessive emotions it is more of a deadening experience. If you put in the same effort in reducing your emotional inputs through the techniques discussed in this book such as Emotional Freedom Technique (EFT) you will experience great highs, joys and emotional release. Through clearing the emotions from your mind-body you will experience far greater highs than any amount of alcohol could provide.

There are a lot of people who drink under the illusion it is relaxing, fun or because it makes them happy etc. This blocking belief is counterproductive if you want to be in great shape. As with food many of the benefits come in the form of false pleasures. They would be much less pronounced if you were already in an emotionally neutral or positive place.

When your life is lacking excitement then drinking may provide that excitement. If your life is already operating on a high level of excitement then you do not need to drink to make it more exciting. If you are unhappy in life then drinking will only ever so temporarily make you slightly less unhappy. If you are truly happy, drinking adds little benefit to the situation.

If you think that drinking makes you happy then just go spend some time speaking with regular drinkers as they tell you their life story. It is very apparent they are far from happy. Alternatively go and stand outside a night club and watch drunk after drunk come out looking miserable, in tears or looking for a fight. They are not happy.

The desire to drink, like any addiction, can also be borne out of a nutritionally based craving rather than any emotional ones. The problem with this is it is almost impossible to tell the difference between a food based craving and an emotional based craving. The only way to know is by seeing what cravings are left once you have got your nutrition in place. When it comes to nutrition a healthy diet is not enough. You must consider aspects such as your calorie intake, ratios of protein: carbs: fat per meal, micronutrients as well as other factors and then see what you are left with. In general almost every addiction is lessened greatly by getting the nutritional elements resolved and almost every addict has failed to get their food right.

Another issue affecting drinking is that it has now become one of the main methods for meeting people and catching up with friends. Though this may be our culture you can still see your friends and not drink. If you feel you have to drink then just have a couple instead of getting wasted. If you combine this with providing other non drinking social events to do then you can really have the best of both worlds.

The more social events you set up away from the drinking scene the better for your results. Try joining a sports club or a society you have an interest in, for example, you could go rock climbing over boozing, a dance class over clubbing, walking over partying, a weekend away instead of a night on the town. If you are reading this and thinking that is boring, then stop and think of something that would not be boring to you. Anyone can go and get drunk every week. It isn't trendy, clever or anything special.

For many people drinking and going out is one of their main strategies for meeting and finding a partner. As mentioned, if you need to be drunk to facilitate the process then you need to develop your confidence so you can do it sober. In today's world of the internet there are now more ways than ever to meet a potential partner that do not need to involve alcohol.

Remember that for many people alcohol is not the major block upon their goals. If it is a problem for you getting into amazing shape then start to investigate the reason behind the drinking and soon you will find the solution.

BLOCKING BELIEF - EATING AND DRINKING TO EXCESS IS FASHIONABLE

This whole concept of taking things to an excess is created from your group dynamics and interactions. Assuming your social group is out of shape then it creates three possibilities that may cause your behaviour to go awry. One is following the group norm which will simply produce bad results. Another is that you may try to beat and supersede others in the group in mimicking their bad behaviours, e.g. trying to eat or drink the most. Finally there is the possibility of generating excitement in your life by rebelling against an expectation, e.g. eating something because you are "not" allowed to.

If all of your peers are out of shape then fitting in with your friends will ensure you also become out of shape. You will be copying their ineffective behaviours that produce poor results. The majority of people in general society are out of shape and suffer from various health issues.

There are many expectations upon you to act badly, overeat or drink. These stem from your friends and family as well as general society. Come Saturday night you may feel a certain social pressure telling you that you should be out partying. You will feel it is the trendy or fashionable thing to do, as it is what everyone else does. If you happen to be staying at home one Saturday night then this expectation may result in making you feel deprived or depressed. Other examples include expectations to eat badly at Christmas, when on holiday or on your birthday. This social pressure may have nothing to do with what you actually want but it will be there affecting you in some way.

Worse than simply following along with the ineffective strategies used by others in your peer group is trying to outdo others in these very same poor behaviours e.g. who can drink the most, eat the worst or be the laziest. Your body would prefer you to compete on things that actually benefit you rather than hurt you. Whichever way you compete it will usually accelerate results which can be as disastrous as it could be beneficial.

The final way social norms trick you into behaviours that are detrimental for your health is by the false sense of excitement they may create when you break from your "healthy living" regime. Wherever we are from and whatever our upbringing we have certain expectations. The voice in your head has the influence of parents, friends, personal experiences and general society within it. When you rebel against an expectation within your mind you will usually create excitement.

Almost all of us have got it implanted in our mind that we shouldn't drink, smoke or eat too much. Therefore rebelling against these thoughts can appear exciting. This excitement is different from looking for more excitement in your life as discussed previously. This excitement is the rebellious voice towards society. It is a self generating excitement, "because I shouldn't do it, it makes it exciting to do, so I will do it!". You feel carefree and a buzz because you are taking a risk by rebelling against what you should not do.

The irony is society no longer cares what you are doing. You are not rebelling against anyone except your own perceived limits. Unfortunately society eats poorly and drinks to excess as a normal behaviour these days. It is deemed acceptable to do this so you are not rebelling, merely fitting into the social norm. You are just being a sheep in society's march to even worse health. You may think 30 million people cannot be wrong. Sadly they can! We once thought the world was flat and cigarettes were good for your health. Our current views on health can be equally absurd.

When you realise that the social norm from society today is a blueprint to be out of shape then you will start to question why are you following the pack when it obviously does not work? If you are rebelling against society, then ask yourself against who and what are you rebelling? What most people are rebelling against is their own beliefs of what they should not be doing.

BLOCKING BELIEF – X, Y, Z IS HEALTHY / UNHEALTHY

Every day we are inundated with statements about healthy living, e.g. bananas are good for you, they contain potassium, onions have high levels of Vitamin C, running is good for you, running is bad for you, this contains phytonutrients, just 2% fat, good fats, bad fats and so forth.

Some of these facts may be true, others not. Our health advice comes as much from the influence of marketers as it does scientific fact. Whatever the credential they are all based on a false model. The assumption is that it is the properties of the external stimulus e.g. food, exercise etc that determines its effect. The reality is that the effect of any food, nutrient or behaviour can only be viewed and analysed in relation towards your body. This is the basis of the statement 'one man's meat is another man's poison". The concept of good or bad in an absolute sense does not exist in the majority of issues surrounding your mind-body.

This is usually hard for people to truly grasp because our society is the other way round. Modern medicine looks at the external stimulus with much greater priority than the internal environment it is introduced to. We see germs, viruses, bacteria and bugs as the causes of our illnesses and not the internal environment of our body and how it deals with these stimuli.

The underlying cause of this upside down approach to health is that the current medical model treats everyone as being the same, whether you are black or white, big or small, left or right brained your body is viewed as being the same as the next persons. The model therefore assumes we all have the same nutritional needs to be healthy.

The problem is as humans we are not all the same. We have great variance on all aspects nutritionally and thus what works for you may not for me. The optimal plan for you to follow may also have little correlation to the typical model of "healthy living"

Therefore, if you rely on any expert that promotes the external stimulus of a food / behaviour without consideration for your internal environment then you may struggle.

People in great shape know that general healthy eating views may not work for them, of course some people in great shape are very well suited to what is promoted as healthy living. However you may not be at all like that person. This is an important concept to grasp. It is irrelevant how many people say something is healthy, whether it is a famous celebrity, a known expert or a Doctor on TV. The only thing that matters is how it affects YOU!

I cover this vital topic in more detail as one of the characteristics of people in amazing shape. In the meantime you need to open your mind on the issue of things being good or bad, healthy or unhealthy in their own right. While certain things may offer no health benefits e.g. smoking, the majority of advice to be healthy or unhealthy is more person specific. This includes eating vegetables, meats, fats, sunlight, exercise and more. For every person where one thing proves beneficial for someone else it may negatively affect their body.

BLOCKING BELIEF - WHEN I DO "A" IT AUTOMATICALLY LEADS TO "B"

We are creatures of habit and often develop an eating reaction to a certain behaviours or events that happens in life. When this is repeated enough times it creates a blocking belief that we have to do this behaviour each time we encounter the stimulus.

Some of the many possible examples include; "I have to eat my two bowls of cornflakes in the morning", "When I go shopping I must have my chocolate bar", "I need that cup of tea when I first get to work", "I have to eat some sugar when I am feeling tired", "I eat chocolate when I am sad", "When John and I go out we always get really drunk", "I have to clear my whole plate when I eat". These statements all suggest that the appearance of one event stimulates or necessitates the reaction. While in some cases this may be true, in the majority it is a something you have simply learned to believe over time.

When a certain behaviour always occurs after another event or stimulus, then assuming it is not by choice, there are three main reasons it happens. This may be because the behaviour has become an anchor, so when one event happens you subconsciously react by doing the second event. Alternatively it is your emotional coping strategy to that situation. Finally it could be you are using this event as an excuse or reason to undertake a behaviour you have 'banned' yourself from doing but a part of you wants to do it.

An ingrained emotional anchor can be a problem. This is because an anchor produces an immediate and often subconscious behaviour. This means you may have eaten your bit of cake the moment you walked in the house while on automatic and without thinking. Anchors will often leave you eating a food even when you do not really want to eat it. You just do it automatically, like one of Pavlov's dogs salivating to the sound of the bell even if it was not hungry.

A way round this is to develop a very negative view of your previous behaviours. If you have a negative view of any behaviour that prevents you being in great shape then your old anchor of eating will automatically be replaced by your new one, which is a strong negative view of your previous behaviour. For example, instead of grabbing that cake when you come in the house you are instead annoyed at the thought of eating junk food and cake because it ruins your body. The new anchor can override the old one.

You will see this effect at work if you notice how ex smokers are often more critical towards smokers than people who have never smoked. The ex smoker needs a strong distaste for smoking so when the anchors kick into place to smoke, it is met by a hatred of smoking which will offset and overpower any cravings.

If you are intent on success it is important to be able to see just how stupid and ridiculous the behaviours that have got you out of shape truly are. For example, let's say the major reason you have a protruding stomach is because of your bread consumption and sensitivity towards it then you should be angry, annoyed and feel negative towards the bread. This is the very food that has made you so unhappy. Most people instead convince themselves they love the bread, chocolate, cakes or whatever else it may be. It is the reason you continue to fail to achieve your goals. People in amazing shape do not love foods that upset their body the most.

When you have an anchor associated to an event you can also begin to break down the anchor by simply changing something. This can be something very small to begin and then increase as you go. For example, if you believe whenever you eat you must clear the plate then you can start by leaving half a fork's worth, then a whole fork and so on until you can eat just what you need. If you eat one brand of chocolate at the supermarket then look to change the brand, then change to another food e.g. from a chocolate bar to biscuits, then to fruit and then to the behaviour needed for success (e.g. not eating at the supermarket). Alternatively just go to a different supermarket.

Anchors are knocked out of balance by any subtle change which removes the direct anchor. In fact many anchors are removed simply by becoming aware of them working on you. In combination with this, look to develop a negative view of that same behaviour. You can do this by looking for negative consequences of the behaviour and repeating these to yourself regularly. This will allow you to crush your anchor for good.

The second reason for a behaviour occurring in response to a certain situation is that it is simply your current choice for emotional management. In this case you need to use better emotional strategies. The size of the emotion experienced will be linked to the severity of the emotional response if it is your emotional coping strategy. This means that you may eat more chocolate after a big argument than for a small argument.

The difference between this and the emotional anchor discussed above is the behaviour will happen only in the presence of an emotion. However, you have to be careful that the regular pattern of using this emotional coping strategy does not form into an anchor itself. For example, if you eat some cake each time you have an argument with your partner, which usually happens when they come home from work then you may find this develops into an emotional anchor that you eat cake every single time they come home from work regardless of whether you do or do not have an argument.

The final reason you may eat rubbish when a certain event happens is if you are using it as an excuse to eat badly or behave wrongly. In this case you may actively seek out the situation or circumstances so that you can then eat whatever foods you want or do the wrong behaviours and be free from guilt because it was not your fault.

I know I have done this myself, I will not eat junk food unless I have no food in the house. Yet, time after time I used to end up with no food in the house! This was especially true if I was under some stress. I realised after a while that this was just my excuse to allow me to eat some poorer quality foods. I was using the 'no food in the house rule' as an excuse to eat some junk food.

If you are thinking "I do this behaviour because I love doing it" then assuming it is a block upon your goals you need to raise the levels of happiness within your life, look for other ways to fulfil the same benefits it gives you as well as continuing to break down the many blocking beliefs outlined here. Arguing you love doing a behaviour that ruins your body is not thinking like someone who is in amazing shape. Remember there are no rights or wrongs when it comes to your beliefs. However, your beliefs will create your results. So if you are not in amazing shape already then you are going to have to change some beliefs or you will continue to get exactly the same results. Believing a negative behaviour on your body is enjoyable can prove a big block to success.

BLOCKING BELIEF – FOOD MAKES ME HAPPIER WHEN I AM HAPPY

Many people have an emotional behaviour pattern where they grab for food or drink when they are happy or as a means to celebrate. This can produce the destructive pattern where you eat both when you are down and when you are up! This invariably ruins your body.

Eating when you are happy has two distinct differences. One is when you eat to celebrate big events, e.g. an engagement, new job, passing your exams, birthdays etc. These are usually infrequent and rarely act as a block on your path to being in amazing shape unless they form into frequent events each week. The other is when you are feeling good on a normal afternoon and then eat to feel "even happier". This will cause greater problems for your goals.

This latter type of eating when you are already feeling happy stems from three main reasons. It could be you are just looking to add more pleasure to an already good situation. The second reason is that being happy could anchor into previous happy experiences which often have been set around food. Finally, eating when you are happy could be an attempt to suppress your emotional stress about past, present or future events.

Eating to add more pleasure to a situation usually stems out of fear or concern that these sorts of events are short lived and infrequent. As a result you try to do as many things as possible to make that situation even better, in case it never comes around again. Liken it a little to me saying you could not eat again for two days, how big a meal would you try to eat before the two day famine? Looking to pile on extra happiness in a situation when you are already happy is little like overeating before a period of no eating.

The problem with this is the food does not add much to the experience and after the initial pleasure feeling has passed you feel worse biochemically. In the end it detracts from the happiness you are experiencing. This is called magnifying happiness. That is the length of time you feel good and happy after an event. You can extend the time you feel happy (magnify) or you can cut it short. Consuming foods that will irritate your body (typical foods we eat for pleasure) serves to cut short your happiness.

You can test this effect for yourself. The next time you are feeling good for whatever reason avoid doing anything to feel even better. Note down how long you feel good for, e.g. twenty minutes, four hours, one day etc. Repeat this when you next feel good but now allow yourself to be 'even happier' by eating the typical foods you use for extra "happiness". Again note down how long the happiness lasts. For most people there will be a big difference in the length of the happiness feeling. You will probably blame the curtailed happiness in the second test on some event that happened in your life to cut it short. Keep trying the experiment though and you will continually find these events cut short your happiness after you eat such foods. This is because food and drink chemically alters your mood. This refers to foods that have a negative effect on your body, which are usually the typical junk type foods you reach for when trying to add happiness to a situation. However, if your normal food curtails happiness then there is a good chance that the meal is not as good for your body as it should be, even if it is 'healthy' by traditional standards.

When you are happy about the elements of your life going the way you want or if you are celebrating bigger news such as a new job, passing a test, a new relationship etc you should learn to enjoy the good feeling. You do not need to go anywhere or do anything as this hides some of the enjoyment of the full experience. It covers up the true emotion in the same way you would try to cover up a negative emotion with behaviours such as eating and drinking. The true feelings of satisfaction and fulfilment will surge through your body in a warm feeling. When something needs celebrating there is already a buzz of excitement in you and usually it is accompanied by a wave of relaxation. You will feel different inside. This is the feeling you want to experience.

To mask this good feeling by eating excessively at dinner, getting drunk or eating junk is depriving yourself of the enjoyment of experiencing the true success you have earned. Instead find a way to amplify your happiness, listen to music, sing, dance, tell your friends / family or whatever actually magnifies the feeling. My definition of magnifying a feeling is to make it last longer and to resonate more within your body. Alcohol and food both shorten the experience and destroys the way the feeling lasts within your mind-body. Over indulging is an awful way to celebrate success!

Many people celebrate happiness with food and drink not because they fear it will not happen again anytime soon but because they are uncomfortable dealing with the good feelings. Being left only with your good feelings can appear very strange and novel at first, but simply relax and enjoy these new feelings before finding ways to magnify it. Watch out for your own expectation that you have to do something. The expectation is simply the pressure of society and your prior conditioning once again.

The second reason you eat when happy is due to anchors as discussed previously. Over the years you will have developed an anchor that says when things go well you should celebrate it with food or drink. This has been implanted by general society and its views. The more you do this behaviour the further it cements and creates a stronger anchor. This means you will return to the behaviour whenever you are feeling good because that is what you do when something is going well, e.g. you treat yourself to that cake, open the wine etc. This layers upon the past and soon you begin to think you cannot enjoy feeling good without food / drink.

The anchors formed by the combination of using food for pleasure while you already are happy can be fairly destructive. They are started young and for no other reason than by your parents copying what their parents did. The result is you will eat food whenever something good happens. Worse than that, we will often return to these same foods when we feel bad and down in a search for that 'lost happiness'. The result is you are eating when you are both up and down which is a disaster for your body. This can be resolved by practicing feeling happy without adding food to the mix and using substitute behaviours.

The final reason you may eat even though you are happy is because the emotions around your mind-body have grown too large. Immediate happiness is related to your present tense evaluation of life. Despite this area of your mind being full of good feelings there are still emotional contributors from events in your past and concerns in the future. This can create enough emotional turmoil (mostly subconsciously) to create the need to use an emotional coping strategy.

The future concerns are especially applicable because you may have received some great news to make you feel good but it may well bring with it uncertainly. Getting a new job will bring the question of how will you resign from your current job, how will you fit in with your new workplace etc. Alternatively, finishing one task at work may make you feel happy but then you have concerns the next task you now have to do is one you really do not like. This excess emotion may push you into using food or drink to suppress these feelings. Dissolving your emotional stress is the best remedy for this and can be effectively done using a variety of techniques which are discussed within this book.

BLOCKING BELIEF – "OLD BILL" LIVED UNTIL HE WAS 90 AND HE DID X, Y, Z

If you recall the definition of being in great shape it went further than simply being about how you looked on the outside. It is equally important to be in amazing shape on the inside! The issue of internal health is one that many people overlook in their obsession to achieve the body beautiful. The reality is that the external appearance of the body is dependent on the internal health. With that in mind any belief that compromises healthy living values can therefore prevent results. This blocking belief is a case in point.

It is common to hear people in bad shape use the example of an old person who did a similar behaviour to justify the habits they know they shouldn't be doing. It is the saving grace of people who live a terrible lifestyle for their body. They can often be found citing the person who lived to 95 who got to this grand age despite drinking, smoking or eating a certain way.

It is fine to idolise someone who has lived into old age. However, we are all unique with our own strengths and weaknesses genetically. It means some of us are more resilient towards aging than others. It is exactly the same situation that we have with 'Fake Thin people'. They are thin despite their efforts, not as a consequence. It is just another example of how special and different we all are as human beings. The question is, how do you know that your genetics are as strong as Old Bill who is still going strong at age 90?

Whenever I hear someone use this ridiculous justification of their behaviours I usually refrain from pointing out those who were not so fortunate. If you look at every person sitting there over 90 years old that smoked there will be many more who died prior to age 60. If you are going to stand behind the old man who is 90 and did X, Y or Z you need to be reminded of all those who didn't make it to 90 who did X, Y or Z.

This is very important because you do not know what your genetic strengths and weaknesses are in comparison to the elder person to whom you are referring. You better hope you have their strength and resilience. Statistically the evidence suggests you will not have their good fortune. This is because we are getting fatter and less healthy. The way your body handles life and your expected health can be summed up from the equation:

(Genetic potential + Positive lifestyle factors) – (Time / aging + Accumulated stressors) = State of health[2]

Your genetic potential is given at birth is your luck of the draw. The medical model believes that this is by far the largest impact on your health. The reality is the factors under your control play a much bigger part than they are given credit for. Even if they were right it promotes an embarrassing state of learned helplessness. This is exactly what we have in our society. Time and aging are also unavoidable but they certainly can go more slowly for some than others due to the way you lead your lifestyle.

Positive lifestyle factors and accumulated stressors are solely under your control. They also form the biggest impacts on your health and appearance. This refers to what you eat, what you do not eat, how much exercise you do, how much you seek out the underlying stressors in your life amongst other things. Anyone who is living to an old age despite doing many an "unhealthy" behaviour will have a strong genetic potential. Whether you have the same strengths it is not known.

When looking at the people who have lived into the upper 80s, 90's and beyond, there can also be confusion over how they got to such grand states. Often when I am hearing stories of how someone lived to a great age the 'bad' behaviours that they cite to justify their own poor personal attitudes to health are no longer applicable. I remember someone saying once "you should have seen the things he drank" yet when I spoke to the elder statesman in question he told me how he hadn't drunk for over ten years. It is common for previous behaviours to be generalised into lifelong behaviours.

The modern world is also a very different environment to what we had in years gone by pollution, poor food quality, excesses of food, a lack of activity, stress, electro-magnetic radiation and spiritual beliefs amongst many other things have all changed over the last 30 years. It means we are facing health issues not previously experienced in the history of mankind. This is why we are the fattest we have ever been as a population.

There can also be confusion about how an older person has lived their life due to our current definitions of what is good and what is a bad behaviour. This issue is very clouded. If you wrongly believe in a one size fits all strategy to health then you may say well my grandmother has eaten full fat products and liver all her life and that did her no harm as you tuck into the cake you just bought.

This argument is not comparable. The grandmother's behaviour is only bad if you subscribe to the fat / meat is bad theory which evidently is not true for a large percentage of the population. Therefore because she did what was actually healthy for her you cannot twist it to justify eating that cake (which you know is not good for you). If you are overweight there is a good chance that the foods in your diet are anything but healthy for you. So saying grandma ate unhealthy foods (when she didn't) to justify eating actual unhealthy foods for you just does not stand up.

Living into old age also has a lot of unseen factors too, including mental outlook which has a massive influence on aging. This cannot be seen from just observing the general eating or drinking habits of a person involved. Your mental outlook includes your emotional stress which is a combination of your spiritual beliefs, evaluation of life and unresolved events from the past. Your emotional stress has a huge influence on your body as does your beliefs about health, internal drive and determination. Have you noticed most people of a grand age are fairly determined, thick skinned and stubborn? They are standing up and fighting aging. The question again of course is, do you have the same mental toughness?

Comparing yourself to older people who have lived to a great age in an effort to justify your behaviours in life is pointless. You should be doing everything possible to help your body and focus on the optimal end of the health spectrum.

BLOCKING BELIEF - I AM HEALTHY ENOUGH.....HEALTH HAPPENS TO ME

Over the years I have met people who were considerably overweight. I have also worked with a long list of clients with various health problems and symptoms. Despite appearing to the outsider as being in a state of poor health I can say I have heard very few (if any) ever say they are unhealthy. Maybe they would say that they live an unhealthy lifestyle but not that their body is unhealthy.

I have lost count of how many times I have heard people say "well, I am healthy enough" as they grabbed their massive beer belly, or "I am perfectly healthy except for my diabetes", "my health is fine but for my asthma", "there is nothing wrong with me but I haven't got much energy" and so forth.

I am perfectly healthy except for ______, is another way of saying I am not healthy. This is important because when people recognise they are not healthy they are usually much more motivated to resolve the problems. This is good because motivated action (with a correct plan) gets results both inside and then on the outside.

I have never really heard people say "I am unhealthy". This is because our flawed medical model basically defines poor health as the inability to move or having a terminal illness of some sort. Possessing a very serious health condition (or not) is the definition most people use for poor health. Therefore people happily fool themselves into thinking they are healthy because they are free from a serious illness. People then wonder why they cannot get into shape because they are "healthy enough".

A more effective view of health would be to use the stages is shown in figure 7:

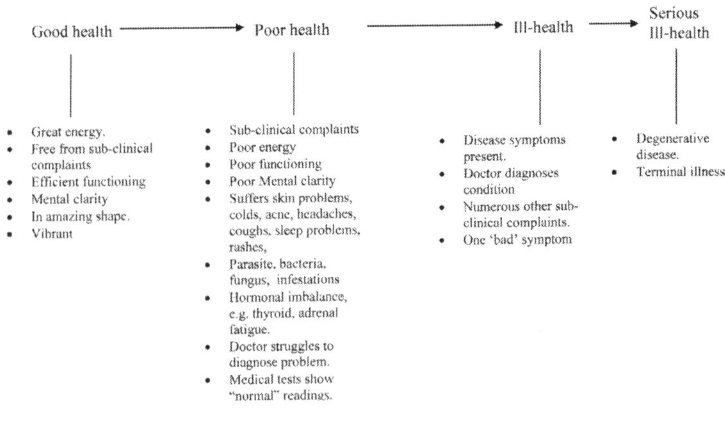

Figure 7 – The four stages of health

What you need to understand is that serious ill-health comes after a stage of ill-health and stems from a period of poor health. When you are using the traditional view of health you will be on risky ground because more often than not you will be fine until you are already in a stage of ill-health. Alternatively you will not feel quite yourself but the doctor is unable to find out what is wrong with you. This is because they use clinical symptoms to diagnose problems. These symptoms usually only appear when you are in a state of ill-health! At this point it is obviously a much greater challenge resolving any condition than when you were in a state of poor or good health.

In regards to getting into shape, the sooner you notice the sub clinical complaints that accompany the poor health stage the sooner you can take responsibility upon yourself to start helping your body way before you need to see a doctor.

The minor headache, the low energy in the afternoon, the skin problem, sleep troubles, frequent illnesses and so forth have all become acceptable parts of normal life. They are acceptable because most people have these traits. Do not believe that makes it normal or ok, most people are overweight. It is not normal for the human body to be overweight. Most people have low energy and a host of health problems.......Do not think it is normal or acceptable!

Between the ages of 5 to 25 years old I had asthma. Like everyone else, I assumed this was fine and felt I was perfectly healthy except for my asthma. I was in reasonable shape and could run fast. The reality was my body was in an awful state and I was in ill-health. I was told there was nothing I could do about my asthma (it was genetic) and I believed it, so I just lived with it. On discovering what my body really needed in order to be healthy I was able to get rid of my asthma and have not needed an asthma spray ever since.

If you are reading this book then I am presuming that you are in a state of at least poor health. If you are saying, "no, my health is fine except for my digestion which is slightly slow and I need to lose 30 pounds (14kg)" then it's important to realise that this is not your optimum health state.

Believers of the genetic theory, which purports to do nothing and instead take a lot of medication, would have you believe you are unable to change this situation. This is false! You have a predisposed genetic need that must be fulfilled, e.g. nutrition, sunlight, environmental factors etc which if not met will result in your body going wrong in a predetermined way. This will be 'your genetics' at play as you are told. For example you may be more likely to put on weight than me but I may develop asthma and allergies. The only question you need to be concerned with is; are you fulfilling your genetic needs? If you are not then you are cheating your body. Remember, following traditional healthy living advice is far from fulfilling your genetic needs to be healthy for most people.

In some people their genetics are the major component of the problem. However, these people are a minority and they would be aware of such medical conditions already. In the vast majority of people their body knows exactly how to be healthy when given the right inputs for their genetics. Therefore the question is - why am I not in the shape I want to be? It comes down to the basics I discussed at the very beginning; your plan of healthy living is wrong or you cannot stick to it or both.

BLOCKING BELIEF - GETTING IN SHAPE IS TOO MUCH EFFORT

The average person can only see effort and hardship in the thought of getting into shape. They may make statements such as "after all this effort, you will probably get hit by a bus" or "life is too short". Everything about getting into shape is too much effort for them. The whole subject of effort is very subjective, what is effort to one person is fine for another and may be enjoyable to a third. What you find an effort one day is enjoyable the next. In general our beliefs about effort in society have contributed to our ever increasing levels of obesity.

In this modern era everything is about reducing the effort needed to do specific tasks. We have escalators to save us walking, remote controls to save us getting up, satellite navigation to avoid using a map, ready meals to save us cooking and home delivery to save the bother of carrying bags. The list goes on and on and on. Each new product aims to reduce the effort involved. Who in the world said that something needs to be less effort for us to do it or enjoy it?

Our obsession with making everything easier in life stems from our beliefs that life is about arriving at the destination and not about the journey itself. Therefore most people get frustrated and annoyed at all the effort they have in their life in the hope of getting to the mystical place of an effort free life, then what? Sit around and watch TV? The beauty of life means that almost everything we do can bring with it joy, interest or pleasure.

When standing in that queue for 10 minutes you can equally use that time to talk to the person next to you, make plans, think about solutions to problems you are having or even do some subtle exercises like breathing technique practice. All this makes life less bothersome and more fun than standing there grunting, checking your watch and moaning how big the queue always seems to be. Every action can be transformed from being an effort to a neutral state but more often than not into a positive event. It is simply a mental outlook game.

Who says it is an effort going to the gym? How can one person love it while another hate it? There are no wrong answers but if you were going to bet on whether someone is going to be in great shape in two years time, who is more likely to get there? The one who thinks the gym is a huge effort or the one who loves it? Why is it a bother to walk to the shops? Who told you cooking every day is a problem? Could it not be a great experience and opportunity to try things? When it comes to things being an effort it is almost always a self fulfilling prophecy, if you believe it to be an effort it will become one and vice versa, if you believe it to be fine, or find ways to enjoy it then it will stop being an effort.

The concept of something being an effort stems from three things, a feeling that you have something else to do, a belief that the task should be easy to do or the thoughts you should not have to do it. These factors will make something feel an effort.

If you believe that you should be at home spending time with the kids then going to the gym will appear an effort. If you think exercising should feel really easy yet you find it a challenge then exercise will again appear an effort. If you feel you should not have to go to the gym or to exercise it will also make exercising a big effort. No wonder getting some exercise done seems so hard with these beliefs running in the back ground. Therefore the key is managing your expectations.

As with almost all our behaviours in life, things being an effort or avoiding something because it is hard is full of contradictions and inconsistencies. In many situations the pain is quite relished. The typical binge drinker takes their hangover in their stride and often jokes about how they had a huge hangover so they couldn't move the next morning. In sport, the participants often enjoy the bruises and minor pains picked up in competition and wear them as badges of honour. Many a gym goer feels cheated unless they have stiffness in their body the next day.

Where is the black and white line between effort, enjoyment and pain? There is no line because we simply choose to believe and make something a good effort or a bad effort. It is another sham that society has taught us that when it comes to health, fitness and getting into shape that everything has to be a bad effort.

If it is ok for you to suffer a hangover for a day why is it not ok to resist a sugar craving? If it is ok to get in early to queue for the January sales then why is it too much effort to queue up for some fresh vegetables? You have no time to cook food yet find time to watch TV, clean the house and do the laundry? It can be easily argued that eating is more important than cleaning your clothes. You will study for a degree for four years yet not take five seconds to study how your body feels two hours after eating. The whole area of effort and pain is a contradiction.

For you to be successful and to be in amazing shape you need to align your views so that the activities that promote success are seen as an enjoyable effort. If it is not, you will be fighting a losing battle against doing the activities. By enjoying the activities that need to be done to create results you will be taking an effortless path towards getting results. The necessary behaviours do not need to be thought of as easy, because some are not, but they need to be thought of as an acceptable effort, something worthy of your persistence and determination. A fun challenge!

BLOCKING BELIEF - WHEN I AM IN SHAPE I WILL FEEL OR BE X, Y, Z

This belief is very much the product of our modern day society and underlies most people's goals to get into amazing shape. It is the cornerstone upon which we base many of our actions and it is the very same reason most people feel unhappy. It refers to the belief that you must attain one thing in your life in order to feel a certain way, e.g. when I have money I will be able to relax, when I am thin I will like myself, when I drive a flashy car others will respect me, when I am in shape I will be attractive and so on.

This premise is based on the belief that obtaining an external object creates a comparable shift internally. This blocking belief goes hand in hand with our model of achievement and the world of celebrity we live in. Everything is about the end result. This sole focus on the end result is because we believe that when you get to your goal there is a pot of gold waiting for you in the form of happiness, self acceptance or achievement. The emphasis on the end reward comes at the expense of understanding the benefits within the journey to get there.

This mistaken thinking pattern is very evident in the world of weight loss. People seek out a specific weight or an ideal body shape and attribute great expectations that will come with it. They are so desperate to get there they try and cheat the process through following crash diets, starving themselves or exercising intensely. This is not experiencing the journey. This is trying to hurry the process so they can get back to doing whatever it was they were doing before. This does not work, to achieve the benefits internally you cannot just change what is on the outside.

To achieve the change internally you need to develop yourself as a person. One way of embracing this journey is asking what feelings are you trying to experience by being in amazing shape? Then think in what ways can you feel those same feelings within your life right now? This will allow you to move faster towards your goals as you will begin to develop yourself in the right areas.

This concept forms the basis of the popular film and book "The Secret" which details the law of attraction. If you feel the way you think you will feel by achieving your goals in the present tense (now), you will be much more likely to go on to achieve your goals. The key is experiencing the emotions now that you wish to feel in the future. This creates a self fulfilling prophecy. To those familiar with "The Secret", I have to point out that most people conveniently forget that it is actions that create results not thoughts. The idea of feeling the way you want to feel is it should lead to doing the actions that will take you there. It is a good thing to think positively, but you must act upon these thoughts. To increase the amount of action you take, increase the amount of emotions you feel when thinking about your goals.

It is important also to look at the reasons you have not achieved your goal. Failure to do so can allow the "I will be happy when I am in amazing shape" belief to occur. If you are out of shape now because you eat when you are unhappy and feel worthless, there is a good chance you hope to achieve your goal weight in order to feel happy and worthy. However, feeling worthy is subjective and a self perception issue. To believe that getting in amazing shape will bring you this feeling is risky business. The journey of getting there could change your views but in general the belief that you are not worthy would contribute to your emotional stress and result in you not sticking to the right eating plan or exercise routine. To overcome this you will need to look at addressing your underlying emotions and in doing as many activities today that make you feel happy and worthy.

In reality this blocking belief is difficult to spot because the way you change internally will often happen simultaneously to your body changing shape. This means it is easy to think the external changes are creating the internal ones. Happiness and being in shape are highly correlated. Therefore it is important to help yourself by finding ways to be happy that do not rely on external successes.

A way to understand this is to think of typical goal achievement being that you hope to get to the goal and thus receive your rewards and benefits. In the real world you go on a journey and by the end of the journey you discover that what you wanted was always inside of you from the outset. However, only the journey allowed you to notice this.

As this is beginning to sound a little philosophical, I will remind you that the body is quite mechanical in terms of getting in shape. Therefore underpinning all this is what you eat, do not eat, exercise etc. However, the ability to do this is tightly linked to the feelings you are experiencing. Feel more of those that you truly desire (why you want to achieve your goal) and sticking to the food and exercise plans long term becomes plausible and realistic. Experience less of these and you become inconsistent and achieve limited results.

BLOCKING BELIEF - I CANNOT DO X, Y OR Z

The statement "I cannot" is a destructive belief to have. It is a phrase that can creep into all areas of your life. This statement will serve to keep you in the place you are now. I have found people who are in poor shape use this statement a lot in the areas of health and fitness. I can't go to the gym today, I cannot start walking in the evenings, I can't eat that food, I cannot give up cereal for breakfast, I cannot find the time to cook and so on. It is one excuse after another. The problem with the phrase "I cannot" is that it leaves no room for behavioural change and closes the mind off from searching for possible solutions.

In my experience people who are overweight love to argue about how they cannot do something. They take such pride in articulating their point, oblivious to the fact their ramblings have become a contributing reason that they cannot change their behaviour and get into shape. Everyone has limitations, stresses and various issues they must battle against if they are to be in great shape. "Argue for your limitations and sure enough they are yours" is a quote from Richard Bach that sums up the overuse of 'I can't'.

This statement is an affirmation which like all affirmations is merely a reflection of your underlying beliefs. The problem with affirmations is they create a catch 22 by keeping you stuck in your current situation which then reinforces your affirmation to be true. Through changing this negative language pattern you will at least open up the avenue for behavioural change as you begin to alter your beliefs. You need to begin questioning every action you do and every action you should be doing.

You can do this by replacing the word "I can't" with "I won't"[3]. The statement I won't (I will not) immediately leads you to the question why not? This is the first step in the process of behavioural change. I won't go to the gym in the mornings....why not? (As opposed to saying I can't go to the gym in the morning...no way!), I will not give up my breakfast cereal....why not? I won't go to the gym 4 times a week....why not? I won't be able to follow a nutrition plan....why not? I won't walk to work....why not? I will not make a vegetable juice every morning....why not? When you answer the "why not?" you will find the reason/excuse that you must overcome to move forwards with implementing new behaviours.

People who live off the I can't attitude like to use statements such as 'it is ok for you but I ____' and 'I know you can do that but I cannot because ____'. When you work with enough people you begin to see that the actual circumstances people cite do not make a difference. I have seen people in similar circumstances both succeed and fail. This includes successful business owners, mothers who have three children, people with a second job, night shift workers etc. These individuals either created the time to get into amazing shape or created the excuses about why they couldn't.

In reality almost every possible work, family, personal or social schedule will allow you to get great results. Likewise, almost every possible schedule will also give you a convenient excuse why you "can't" do what you need to do. The real tragedy is that very often it is not an excuse that prevents you it is simply that you never thought of doing it differently, this is often the case and is one of the reasons why saying "I can't" is so destructive. The language prevents you questioning the behaviour or looking for a better solution. Change "I can't" to "I won't" and see how many solutions your mind creates.

Another issue of 'I can't' is the overall belief that you cannot achieve your goals. To be successful you do not need to believe you can succeed. There are millions of people who can act as testimonials who have achieved something despite never believing it is possible. However, your beliefs need to be open minded enough to try. Actions create results so as long as you do what is right there is no need to believe in the first instance that you will be successful. The problem most people have is they do not engage in the necessary behaviours unless they believe they will ultimately be successful. It is the lack of actions not beliefs that stops results.

Applying the 'I won't' to 'I can't' on your overall success opens up the question of why won't you get into amazing shape? This will be enough to get things moving, e.g. If the statement 'I cannot lose three stone' becomes 'I will not lose three stone' which opens the question why not? If the answer is "Because I have no will power!" The solution is to start developing your mind set before trying to get in shape.

BLOCKING BELIEF - BEING HEALTHY COSTS TOO MUCH MONEY

The perception that being healthy costs too much money is one made up by a society that puts more emphasis on nice possessions than a flourishing mind-body. I have lost count of how many people driving nice cars complain about the price of the food, fitness training or similar. I have met many people who have just spent hundreds of pounds on clothes yet won't find the money to aid their body. People on a budget find it more acceptable to spend money on alcohol, junk food and cigarettes than to spend it on sorting out their health.

As a society we have the cheek to not only expect the body to look after itself for free but then we go on and abuse it in every way possible. We complain when our body goes wrong yet we fail to take it for a service even after years of abuse. It is strange how most people will take their car in for a service each year yet would never spend time maintaining and fixing their own body. If your car breaks down you do not expect the mechanic to sort it for free, yet when it comes to personal health, anything that's not free is perceived as being costly.

Getting in to great shape is an investment, just like a car or house is an investment of your money. For people on a budget they can still achieve their goals. It does not cost the earth to get in great shape when you know how to do it. The problem most people have is not the actual cost but the priorities they hold. The amount of money I see spent on the likes of designer clothes, bags, shoes, drinking, cigarettes, gambling and more is senseless. These are often the individuals that think they cannot afford to be in great shape.

The internet is awash with free information on exercise and nutrition, organic foods are decreasing in price, learning the basics of most behaviour change techniques can be done for free online, doing exercise in the park is free. There is so much you can do without spending much money. Cost should never be the blocking factor to obtaining success. For most people it is just another excuse. If budget is an issue what free or low cost things can you do to help your body?

BLOCKING BELIEF - EATING FAT MAKES YOU FAT

This is one of the most prevalent blocking beliefs today. How many people were fat in the 1950's and 1960's? The answer is dramatically less than today, yet fat consumption, especially saturated fat was consumed in greater amounts fifty years ago than the present day. If you look into data about fat consumption you will find that there is not the correlation with body fat levels[4] that we have been led to believe.

As we have become fatter we have consumed less fat as a society. Ask yourself this, how many low fat diets have you been on? (Bear in mind that typical healthy eating is a low fat diet) yet what results have you got? Do you think it is strange that as the fattest society in the history of mankind we are also the only society to have eaten low fat?

Like so many 'facts' on nutrition the issue of fat is messed up. This is why relying on facts put forward by the government, medical community or similar to get you in shape may leave you facing a long drawn out struggle. Whatever your body is like there is a good chance your body thrives on fat. We are designed to eat it. There was no low fat when your ancestors lived in the wild. Through avoiding it you are depriving the body of vital nutrients which may conversely result in you being overweight.

This doesn't necessarily give you the green light to go and eat unlimited amounts of fat based foods. But neither should it mean you avoid it within the diet. The key is to find the threshold that work for you.

BLOCKING BELIEF - BUT IF EVERYONE DID THAT THEN......

This is a phrase I have heard more times than I care for. It comes in the form of "if no-one drank the world would be a boring place", "if we couldn't go out and eat how would we all catch up", "the food industry wouldn't exist if we all followed your recommendations".

These generalisations are another subtle excuse given out. Let's be honest, the world is not going to change dramatically overnight. There will always be people who continue the very behaviours you need to change away from. There will always be people who think food makes them happy, those who think they are rebelling against society by drinking and others who have no alternative strategies to quash their emotions but to eat.

The changes you make will not affect the situation. The world will go on without you eating a bag of sweets, or getting drunk, or smoking etc. You will experience an initial disruption in your life but it will only be a small ripple and everyone around you will soon adapt.

It's important not to live off this false view of the world. People have undue beliefs of grandeur by how important their behaviour is to a situation. The truth usually is that your behaviour is just a slight influence and the same situation will continue, your friends will still be friends, your family will still love you and you can still win the business contracts, promotions in work and any other excuse that you give for why you must eat or drink to fit in with the world.

BLOCKING BELIEF - CALORIES

The issue of calories and their role in losing fat is a subject for much debate within the field of nutrition. Like many theories with two sides arguing the complete opposite to each other, the truth usually lies somewhere in the middle.

Pure calories subscribers claim it is all about that magical calorie number and nothing else whereas anti calorie proponents feel that calories are irrelevant and it is the types of food that determines your success.

I have spent time subscribing to the calories only approach and also being against calories. I now sit firmly in the middle with the understanding both sides of the debate are right.

The reason this is important for you is that the more firmly you sit at either end of the spectrum the more it will compromise your level of results.

The calories theory has it right in regards that you need to consume fewer calories than your body needs to lose fat. It is also helpful as most people have no idea about what is in food or how much of that food they are eating.

The non-calorie approach has it right in that foods affect your body differently in both terms of health and fat loss. There will be some foods that lead to fat gain more quickly than others.

Where the calories approach falls down is assuming our calories needed per day are set in stone at a certain level, in its assumption a calorie deficit necessarily is made up by using your fat stores and the idea all calories are created equal at the expense of considering their roles within your body.

The non-calories approach fails in that it does not explain the mechanism of fat loss nor explain why you could take any person, lock them in the cell and give them a very low calorie diet of any food and they would lose fat. They would feel awful but they would stay alive and lose fat regardless of food type.

Pure calorie subscribers like their theory because they can eat any food as long as calories are accounted for. A problem though is most people do not count calories when they are being "bad". Non-calorie subscribers like their theory because they do not have to monitor how much they eat as long as it is the right food. Their problem is they ignore the times they eat the wrong foods.

The key for you is dropping the element of the belief that is preventing success. If you are counting calories rigidly then you may need to examine the content of these calories and the accuracy of your counting. Conversely, if you have no calorie awareness you will most likely not be aware of how much you actually consume or know how much your body needs.

BLOCKING BELIEF - THE POWER OF FREE FOOD AND LINKING FOOD TO MONEY

The power of 'free' is an effect that has been studied in business circles as it has a disproportionate response from consumers[5]. When the word 'free' is bandied about you will see people clamouring to get some of the free goodies before they are all gone. People will not evaluate the issue about whether they actually want the product because they are gripped by the fear the free stuff may be gone when they have finally made their decision.

When it comes to food this clamouring for a free lunch can overrule many nutritional principles. I know this from personal experience. By saying no to free food you feel you are losing out on money because you could have had something for nothing and you do not want to wait around in deciding in case someone else takes it.

The reality is that your body does not know the price tag of food. It does not care whether it was free or if you paid £1 or a £1000. The body will judge it on the same level whatever the case may be. The body simply digests the food, absorbs what it needs and handles the toxins that may be present and adjusts body fat levels as it sees fit.

This also applies when you go to a restaurant. You pay for your meal and endeavour to finish your meal so you can be sure you get value for money. The truth is you have paid your money whether you finish it or not. It makes no difference. The restaurant will dispose of whatever you leave and you will be no richer by finishing it. The only thing you get for forcing yourself to finish a meal is feeling more bloated than if you stopped when you felt full. You never get your money back and nor does the restaurant make any more money from you if you leave some of your meal.

You can see the association of money to food in many situations. These include restaurants, business lunches, food passed around the office, foods you have bought etc. It is important to break any connection that links what you eat to money as this can lead you astray. The most economical way to view and handle food is to eat until full then save the rest for later. Understand that in situations where this cannot happen you gain nothing by trying to eat everything.

BLOCKING BELIEF - FINISH YOUR PLATE THERE ARE STARVING CHILDREN IN AFRICA

This is what most parents tell their children growing up in order to get them to finish their meals and it is one of the childhood beliefs that stick with us as adults. Once food has been served up on your plate it is considered used. Therefore whether you eat it or not, it will not be of use to anyone else. It is unrealistic to think you are going to send your leftovers by post to Somalia. It has no bearing on kids in Africa. Once it is on your plate it is used. In fact, you could argue once it is even in the country it is used produce. Therefore the way to reduce food intake is to cook and eat only what you need at that time and to save the rest for another meal time.

Even if everyone in the West did finish what was on their plate it will have little effect on the food issue in Africa. The world has enough food to sort that problem out now if it wanted to. It is a huge political / logistical crisis that prevents it from happening. So put aside any self reasoning that what's on your plate affects their situation.

Reducing overall food consumption is never a bad thing though as it lessens the demand we place on our environment. To individually reduce your food consumption, look to become completely accustomed to not finishing food on your plate. I actively practice this behaviour by rarely finishing a plate of food. I eat what I need and move on then and leave the rest for later.

Many people finish their plate in an attempt to control their hunger. Though it may appear a sensible way to stave off that hunger feeling the best way to control it and reduce consumption of foods is to give your body all that it needs within a meal by using the right amounts of protein to carbohydrates to fats. This will reduce hunger for maximal durations and allow you to reduce your overall consumption while also feeling great!

BLOCKING BELIEF - IT TAKES TOO MUCH TIME TO BE IN SHAPE

The reality of achieving your goals is that it takes much less time than people think it should and when you enjoy what you need to do to be successful you will easily find the time anyway. It does require some time on your part but I always maintain it takes up more of your time being out of shape, having low energy and suffering from poor concentration than it does by committing the time to resolving these issues.

When it comes to time commitment many people confuse the requirements of being a professional athlete with the requirements to be in great shape. Being a professional athlete is a full time occupation. Being in amazing shape is something everyone can achieve with a moderate time investment. If creating your sensational body is mostly about losing fat then most of this is determined by how well you eat and not how much time you commit to exercising etc. As everyone needs to eat, you can easily find the time to make sure you eat well for your body. It is just as simple to eat well as it is to eat badly.

If your current availability of time to get in shape is actually less than the minimal amount needed to be successful then you must change your priorities and / or multi task, e.g. combine family time with exercising etc. When it comes to the time factor it usually means your health and fitness goals are simply not high enough in your list of priorities. In some people they simply use a lack of time as a convenient excuse to justify why they are not succeeding. As with all excuses, they never change the result, they simply make you feel a little less worse about failing.

BLOCKING BELIEF - IT IS HARD TO MAINTAIN RESULTS / WHAT IF I PUT THE WEIGHT BACK ON?

Maintaining results is only difficult if the method you achieved them by was using will power and unsustainable behaviour patterns. If you actually get to your goal through natural motivation and accurate subconscious behaviour patterns you will easily stay where you are and enjoy every single moment of it. It is much harder getting into shape than it is to maintain your results. So once you have achieved it in a sustainable way the rest will be easy and manageable!

Fear of loss of face in the event that you fail to maintain the results you achieved is a common fear. The nature of health and fitness is that if you do it in the right way you will never go back. However, let's pretend you did. Most people admire someone who achieved their goal as opposed to someone who has never achieved that goal. Who do you respect more, a person who made a million pounds and then lost it or someone who never made any money?

It is always much better to achieve something and enjoy those benefits (even for a short while) than to never achieve it. It is an invigorating and joyful experience when you are getting results. This awesome feeling is more than worth it even if you were to revert to your original body shape. It is always better to do something than nothing.

The final point to note is that this belief shows that you want to be in shape. Whether you are too scared to go for it or not, it does not change the fact you really want to achieve it. Life is always better when you chase your dreams whether you achieve them or not. This is because working on your goals and dreams is an inspirational behaviour which aligns itself with the third tier of happiness – fulfilment.

BLOCKING BELIEF - I AM OVERWEIGHT BECAUSE I HAVE AN UNDERACTIVE THYROID

This is a classic example of the medical model causing someone to have a state of learned helplessness. A low thyroid is not the reason you are overweight. A low thyroid is simply the symptom of your body reacting to past treatment. As a result the hormonal system has been irritated and your thyroid gland has become diminished.

The real reason you are overweight is the same reason why your thyroid gland has become fatigued. As your body accumulates more stresses during your life from nutritional, physical and emotional sources it takes its effect on the body. If the stresses continue over a prolonged period the body will suffer and other problems may occur one of which includes weight gain and also low thyroid function.

This raises the question, are you going to get to the root cause and restore the health and function to your body or are you going to continue to blame low thyroid as the reason you are out of shape? Blaming your body on any causes that cannot be resolved is a poor excuse. Even if low thyroid activity was the cause of your weight gain, what are you going to do about it?

No health condition should stop you trying to help your body as much as you can. The protocol is the same whatever symptoms you may have. You must eat the right foods, avoid the wrong ones, exercise correctly and remove the underlying stressors within the body. If not, then you are never going to get in shape anyway. Stop using low thyroid activity as the excuse why you are overweight. It is merely a symptom of the real cause.

BLOCKING BELIEF - YOU DO NOT NEED TO LOSE ANY WEIGHT – YOU LOOK GOOD AS YOU ARE NOW

A sure sign you are on the road to success is when people say you do not need to lose any more fat / weight. Remember most people in society are overweight and would not realise what an ideal body fat level looks like. So when you start to get into amazing shape you will start to receive these comments. There are two main points to consider in regards to this issue.

The first element is about knowing what your ideal goal is. In this day and age of more eating disorders than ever before you must know what your ideal body fat percentage is and where you are now in relation to it. In general, if your body fat reading is 10% for men, 20% for women and you are not happy with your body fat then the issue is in your head. Your ultimate goal may be lower than these numbers but you should still be happy about where you are at these levels. I personally vary between 8% - 12% most of the time. When I hit 8% people often say I am too thin. If you veer below 5% for men or 15% for women then this is deemed "medically" to be too low and health problems may occur, e.g. stopped periods, bone density loss etc. If you do not think you are too thin at this level then it could be a measurements issue (inaccurate reading, measurement protocol) or an issue within your mind.

Assuming you are not below 5% (15% for women) then it is important that you know where you are in terms of your goal. It is destructive to let other people influence you with their judgements on your body. Often you can be in receipt of contradictory opinions which can undermine your confidence.

You must know where you are in terms of your goals. You need to know what your goal is, where you are now in relation to it and your progression towards it, then other people's opinions are just that! Opinions! One person's view of what looks good may vary greatly from another persons. Some people are intimidated by your success and may simply try to upset you. Some make statements based on comparisons to other people while certain people may be concerned for your health.

The main thing you need to do is separate fact from opinion. Fact is your current body fat / clothes size, your ideal goal and your current progress towards it. Opinion is how good you look, how someone thinks you should look and how someone thinks they should look etc.

SECTION 3

TEN PRINCIPLES OF HOW PEOPLE IN AMAZING SHAPE THINK

In the last section you learnt about the many lies and blocking beliefs we tell ourselves and hear from society. Each of these serve to keep you stuck exactly where you are and make you both overweight but also unhappy about being overweight. By understanding the impact of these beliefs and their effects on your behaviour you can begin to remove them from your mind. As you do this you will have made it much easier on yourself to get results. However to be in amazing shape you must also begin to think and act like these people do.

When it comes to getting in great shape you will find that successful people share certain key characteristics and thought patterns. There are ten major patterns and characteristics that they hold. These thought patterns mean they automatically behave in a way that produces results. If you want to be in amazing shape too then you will need to adopt these thought patterns.

Within the ten characteristics, I have clearly outlined the differences between people in sensational shape and people in awful shape. These differences are not good nor bad, right or wrong, they are simply a matter of fact. You can either choose to adopt the attitudes the people in amazing shape have or you can take the opposite point of view. Make up your own mind in relation to the issues but the result is that one point of view pushes you towards looking great on the beach while the other will have you looking for winter holidays to hide away under your thermals.

I identified these traits through observing the behaviour of people in amazing shape and comparing the differences between people who succeed and those who fail to get results. This applies to both men and women. I am drawing on experience from those I had the pleasure of meeting in gyms all over the world, from my work with hundreds of clients looking to achieve their goals and those I have met in daily life. I contrast this with the even greater numbers of people I have met who are in poor shape.

Almost every person with a fantastic body will possess each of the ten attitudes in some form and to some degree. Assuming you are not in amazing shape now, the best way to ensure success is to adopt each one of the ten strategies, behaviours and thought patterns that have been observed in people who have flat stomachs, great muscle tone and are confident about their looks. The ten principles are not arranged in any order of importance.

PRINCIPLE 1 – DESERVE SUCCESS AND AVOID SELF SABOTAGE

People in amazing shape are clear about the fact they deserve to be successful and they know it is their right to be in the best shape possible. When you truly believe you deserve your dream body you will stop using your weight as a covering issue for other problems in life and you eliminate self sabotage from your behavioural patterns.

Believing you deserve to be in amazing shape is critical to success. You will not find a millionaire who does not think he deserves to be rich and you will not find someone with a body to die for who thinks they do not deserve to look sensational.

This principle of deserving to be in amazing shape is linked to your feelings of worthiness. It influences your likelihood to self sabotage and goes hand in hand with whether you are using your problems of getting into shape as a covering issue for facing another problem.

Worthiness

How worthy you feel links into whether you deserve success and consequentially to achieving your goal. There is not an objective scale of worthiness. It is a self perception issue derived in your mind based on your prior experiences in life. At birth you are neither worthy nor unworthy of anything that awaits you in life. This remains the case at age 80. The problem is that you may have convinced yourself that you now have a specific ceiling of achievement within different areas of your life and that there are some things you do not deserve to achieve.

You can see your worthiness in the area of money quite clearly. Some people say they are worthy to receive lots of money yet will conversely give you a present they deem is too expensive for their own perceived level of worthiness (believing they do not deserve it). In weight loss this same issue is seen in the way people try to deflect comments about how they are looking good, slimmer etc with common rebuffs such as "It must be the clothes I am in", "you are just saying that".

When you do not feel 100% worthy of getting into shape then you may find yourself allowing obstacles to get in your way. You may think it is not right to dedicate time to get results, you may say it is more important to dedicate your time to something else. You will refuse to see yourself as thinner than other people or in better shape. You may feel being in amazing shape is not for you, it is only for other "different" types of people. When you do not feel you deserve success you will feel uncomfortable in your body as you begin to get results. At the heart of this uncomfortable feeling is a voice saying 'this isn't you', 'you do not deserve this' 'how can you be thinner than your sister' and so on. People in amazing shape know it is their birthright to be in good shape.

The reason people do not feel worthy is because of their prior conditioning and unresolved specific events from the past. Unfortunately the mind is not as logical as it should be. If you feel you did something wrong in your life then you may inflict punishment on yourself by preventing success in the areas you care about the most. This is not logical but it is how the mind works.

The whole concept of worthiness is haphazard. There are many people in amazing shape who do not feel worthy in life. Instead they use this as a motivator to get into shape, to prove they are worthy. If you cannot channel this feeling as a motivator then the good news is you can still achieve the results you desire irrespective of this. Just shift your lack of worthiness to affect another area of your life.

Everybody deserves to be in awesome health. If you were not then why is your body programmed to be in amazing shape? Give it the right stimulus and you will achieve a ridiculous body transformation. This is because your body does not have any preconceived ideas about being worthy.

It reacts to what you do and it has a natural blueprint to take things forward.

In order to feel worthy of success there are a couple of strategies you can follow. One is just acknowledging you deserve it. For this we always look for external validation, maybe your partner, your mother, your father etc. In reality you do not need anyone to tell you this, worthiness comes from the inside not the outside. Most people wait and wait hoping to be told that they deserve to achieve their goal. You will normally be waiting a long time to be told this. Instead tell yourself you are worthy of absolute success, and that you can achieve anything you set your mind to. Tell yourself this today, tomorrow and every day for the rest of your life. The concept of needing to feel worthy is so illogical. At what point in your life did you become worthy or unworthy? As a new born baby were you worthy of success then? How about a 5 year old? 10 years old?

If you still need someone to validate that you are worthy then you are in luck. I have worked with many people and would consider myself perfectly suited to know if you deserve to have an amazing body, great energy and confidence. I can officially declare:

"You deserve to achieve your goals
You deserve to be at your goal weight
You deserve to be free from aches, pains and any health complaints

You deserve to happy, confident and free within your body

You are a great person, you deserve to love yourself, be at peace with yourself.

You are a special person and it is your right to be in amazing shape."

By now you should have realised that you are worthy of success and the whole concept of worthiness is false. It is a myth created in your own mind. No one is worthy or unworthy of realising their goals. Remind yourself that you deserve to achieve your goals and that your body is naturally programmed to be in awesome shape.

As well as acknowledging the self imposed limitations of the unworthiness concept you should also work on the emotions that created this feeling in first place. This can be from previous emotional events or key beliefs that create this feeling.

Self sabotage

Almost everyone who has struggled with achieving their goals understands the principle of self sabotage. There are different reasons you may engage in self sabotage and you may do it to different degrees of severity. One of these stems from a lack of self worthiness as discussed above. Other reasons though include a fear of success, a contradictory goal or a negative experience associated with the last time you were looking your best. Self sabotage can also be linked to will power methods of getting in shape and a drop off in conscious thought.

Fear of success

For people in great shape it is hard to imagine what fears anyone could hold about looking amazing. They think, how can you fear feeling good about yourself each time you look in the mirror? How do you fear having the ability and confidence to do exactly what you want?

To the average person who is not yet in amazing shape they have very real fears about obtaining success. Some common fears people have about being in shape includes receiving unwanted attention off the opposite sex, being unable to maintain results or looking stupid if you put the weight back on. Other fears include other people expecting you to do things differently, losing popularity with friends, changing as a person in a bad way or being singled out.

These fears are ill founded. There is no greater feeling than being in awesome shape and the benefits far outweigh any negatives. In fact, I cannot think of any negatives.

The vast majority of fears are in your head and made up. Many of your fears are no more likely to happen if you are at your goal weight than where you are now. In fact, many of your fears are much less likely to happen if you were in amazing shape compared to where you are now because of the person you will become.

Many people fear that being in shape brings with it a pressure to continue to stay in shape. In reality everyone who is trying to change their body has already put themselves under a tremendous amount of pressure while in the pursuit of their goal. The pressure to maintain results is child's play compared to their current levels.

Putting weight back on is only ever possible if you used questionable methods to achieve it in the first place. Otherwise, why would you put it back on? If your mind set is changed and your plan is correct yet still open to adaption it is very unlikely you will lose weight and then regain it. This book focuses upon making it possible to break the yo-yo dieting process. If you found yourself gaining a couple of pounds then you simply need to revert to focussing your mind set or if the body has changed then you must adapt the plan you follow.

Fearing you may have to act differently is another unfounded fear. It is hard to impart to people who are not in amazing shape how you will be different as a person when you have achieved your goals. You can handle situations with a new confidence, carry out more tasks and in a way where it feels fun and effortless.

It is a common concern that your friends may treat you differently out of jealousy or that you may be singled out. This only ever happens if you lose the weight without developing as a person. Someone truly in great shape does not need to broadcast this, the body speaks for itself. If you respect people and support others you will only become more popular because you will be a nicer and happier person to be around.

Some people feel they will receive unwelcome sexual advances. These fears are linked to confidence. When you go through the process of getting into shape you have to face many hurdles and challenges. These successes develop your confidence and concurrently your ability to handle these situations.

In short almost every fear you have about achieving your goal has not accounted for who you will be when you have achieved it. This version of you will be able to handle these problems effortlessly.

Negative experiences in past

Self sabotage can also result because of unresolved emotions from specific events that happened in the past. If you had something bad happen to you when you were last in great shape then it is likely that you will have negative emotions surrounding a return to that state. This could be that there was an unwanted sexual advance, you were bullied, or something unrelated to your weight happened, e.g. someone died. This will cause you to associate in your mind a negative emotion with being in shape. These specific events contribute to your emotional stress as well as acting as a huge negative anchor for success. The emotions from these events can be reduced using the various emotional reduction strategies (see principle four for more on this).

Contradictory goal

Many people self sabotage not because of a lack of worthiness or fear of success but instead because they simply have a contradictory goal. If your goal is to get in shape so you do not need to worry about anything you eat then you have created a self sabotaging circle. The moment you feel or look good it will give you the green light to go eat whatever you want, which will usually be some sort of junk food. You will do this until you become unhappy with your shape again and then the good eating and exercising kicks back in. If your goal to get into shape is to allow you to eat as much as you want without a care in the world you will forever struggle to be in amazing shape. It is a contradictory goal, it is like aiming to give up smoking so you can then get to the point where you can smoke as much as you want without worrying about it. In such cases you need to review and adjust your motivations for success.

Will power collapse

This common form of self sabotage is not really self sabotage but more the collapsing of an unsustainable behavioural pattern. If your plan to get in shape is based on willpower then it is simply a matter of time before you stop following it. This may seem like self sabotage but it is more a natural wearing down of your efforts. As you see some success you say to yourself "Phew. That was a lot of effort, now I can relax a little because I am making progress". If you want to get into amazing shape and stay there long term you cannot view your health and fitness behaviours as an effort. Everything needs to become natural and something you want to do. This relates to your subconscious beliefs and not your conscious thoughts (willpower).

Using your weight as a covering issue

Failing to achieve your goals can come from a lack of worthiness to deserve success or from one of the different methods of self sabotage stalling your progress. For some people though the reason they do not achieve their goal is that they are using their weight as a covering issue to avoid addressing a different aspect of their life.

When your goal of getting into amazing shape is a covering issue you will usually have an unnatural obsession with trying to achieve it. You will think about it all day long, worry, obsess and panic that things are not going right. Despite all this mental activity you will still find yourself doing behaviours you know you shouldn't do. When progress is made towards your goals you will often manage to find a way to do some crazy moments of self sabotage. The reason for this is that your health and fitness goal has become a distraction to avoid facing another issue. Therefore as you progress it makes the prospect of facing that fear greater than before. You therefore either do nothing to achieve your goal or sabotage your previous progress. This is all at the same time as being obsessed about achieving this same goal.

Self sabotage at this level is very indistinguishable from people who are simply holding a fear of success. Some clues that it is a covering issue include not being happier as you progress towards being in great shape and the answer to the question, "If your body was not an issue in your life, what would you have to do or face up to?"

Obsessions over weight can be used to avoid facing various issues. It could be about the meaning of life or what happens after death. It could be you are avoiding facing a family issue or trying not to think about the state of your life. This includes money, career, relationships and much more. Other people obsess over their goal to avoid thinking about things that have happened in their past.

In these situations your mind-body has created an obsession which is easier to handle than facing up to a greater emotional pain. Your mind-body is really asking for a respite from your deeper thought patterns. It is not about losing weight. In these situations, if you release the mind and the emotions about the underlying issue you will effortlessly go on to achieve your goals.

Whatever the underlying emotional reason may be it will not go away any time soon unless you start using an emotional management strategy. The underlying emotional issues are different to normal emotions experienced because not only are they big issues but they almost always appear to have no way to be resolved. For example, answering questions about the meaning of life and death seems to be an issue that cannot be resolved. However, the numerous emotional management strategies can reduce and ease these emotions.

You can try to shift your obsession to another area of your life to allow you to get into shape. However, it is not easy to shift an obsession because it has developed over many years. One way to adjust the obsession within the area of health and fitness is to try to develop your ability within a sport rather than everything being about getting into shape. The great thing about sports is you can always further obsess about achieving a higher level of performance because you can always get faster / better. Even if you break a world record! It also forces you to rest as much as you train and thus avoid overtraining. Fitness is the balance of training versus recovery, to get fitter you must rest more as you train more.

The best approach inevitably is a combination of both. Removing the emotions from the underlying events can take a period of time so directing the obsession to a more productive area for your body will give you breathing space as you work on the emotions.

Judging your body

A sign that you are using your weight as a covering issue for something else can be seen in how you are able to judge your body. If you currently need to lose a stone of fat (14lbs / 6.5Kg) to be looking amazing then after you have lost half a stone of fat you should feel great! You know you are looking so much better and you feel it too.

However, someone who is using their goal as a covering issue will not feel great. Instead they will obsess about the fact that they haven't lost the other half stone. They will wonder why it is taking so long, what is wrong with them, if only they could lose half a stone more.

The reason you do this is that you do not feel any better. The logical thought process is that you will feel better when you are half way to your goals. However, as weight loss is simply a front for another issue you are avoiding, the progress you have made with your weight makes no changes to this issue and thus you feel no better. Therefore you theorize that it must be because the benefits come only when you hit your magic "goal weight". The truth is you will only make progress by addressing the real issue, when you do that you will feel different and this will allow you to go on to effortlessly achieve your goal and be able to acknowledge it when you are there.

When weight is a covering issue you will also have a total inability to judge your own body with any degree of realism.

This is because your emotions are not coming solely from the judgement of your body. In these situations you see the strange dichotomy in abilities of self evaluation. On the one hand the person is able to spot even the most subtle gains in weight yet also have an inability to notice significant losses of half a stone (7lbs /3kg) and more.

People in great shape know clearly where they are body fat wise. They know what shape they are in and where they should be. If their body changes they are quick to acknowledge improvements. They celebrate and rejoice at the progress they have made. They take this energy and good feeling to drive them onwards further and further. If they have gone slightly backwards they stop and think, what do I need to do to revert this trend? Why has it happened? They look at it from a calm position yet apply focused and concentrated motivation to resolve the issue.

When weight is a covering issue then even those who do go onto achieve their goals will often just move the goals posts. On getting to their goal weight they still feel similar (because the underlying issue is still there) so they then decide that the goal posts must be moved. Now the goal is yet more weight loss, another dress size down. This cycle will continue until the underlying issues are resolved.

Linked to this is ensuring your goal is physically possible for the body shape that you have. While you want to look your best, be lean and toned you cannot change your bone structure. You must make sure that your goal is focused on what you can change over what you cannot. If you hate elements of your body that cannot be changed, e.g. height, bone structure, you must work on your emotions of acceptance. There are many different ways people can look amazing whether you are short, tall, slender or on a larger frame. Your goal should be to look sensational within the structure you already have.

BEHAVIOUR CHANGE EXERCISES

The behaviour change exercises at the end of each chapter use a five step behaviour change process. When questioning your behaviours always look to hold an observational and forgiving attitude rather than a critical or berating view of your current behaviours. Every behaviour you are currently doing (or not doing) serves a specific purpose and it is the best solution you have come up with under your current circumstances, knowledge and skills. There is no point in beating yourself up about it. Simply observe, learn and develop.

With the emotional management section of the five step process you will use various techniques to induce changes at an emotional level. These may range from creating anchors to Emotional Freedom Technique (EFT). These are discussed in a little more depth in principle four. For now just follow along and see how it affects you.

Awareness –

Answer the questions below to reveal some possible beliefs that may need addressing. The answers to these are often quite well hidden and come from deeper within your mind.

Why are you not worthy of being in amazing shape?

If you were not obsessing about your weight, what other issues in life would you have to think about or need to face?

What are your main fears about achieving your goals and being successful?

What are the benefits of being overweight and out of shape?

What types of self sabotage do you use?

Questioning –

Spend some time reviewing your answers from the awareness section. What would it take for you to change your beliefs over to those that support you? Most people are more motivated to achieve things for other people than for themselves. Who would benefit from you being successful in your goal? Who could you help if you were in amazing shape? Who would you inspire? Use this information to motivate you.

Intention

Decide today that you are worthy of success and you deserve to be in amazing shape. Stop using your weight as a covering issue and commit to dissolving the underlying issues underneath this smoke screen.

Touch your hand on your heart and say out loud ten times:

"I deserve to be in amazing shape"

Planning –

Identify the cause of your self sabotage patterns. Make a plan of action to avoid this happening in future occasions.

Emotional management –

Emotionally accept that you deserve to be in shape and let go of your fears. Collapse your main fears about being successful using Emotional Freedom Technique. (Go to www.benwilsonuk.com for an example EFT video). Insert your own fears and concerns into the sentence below as appropriate:

"Even though I fear ______ if I lose weight I accept deeply and completely accept myself"

e.g. "Even though I fear people will be nasty to me if I lose weight I deeply and completely accept myself"

PRINCIPLE 2 – BE INSPIRED BY YOUR GOAL AND GIVE IT EQUAL PRIORITY AS OTHER GOALS

The kind of people who can strip down into their swim wear on the beach and look fantastic will all say the same thing that being in awesome shape is vitally important. It is central to their goals in life and something that they not only deeply care about but find they are inspired by the thought of chasing after it. As they are inspired by their goal it becomes very important to them. This is a significant attitude to hold.

When it comes to goals there are rarely any rights or wrongs, just choices you make which either help or hinder you towards your success. How important you view your goal is an attitude that can greatly influence how many of the behaviours you choose to do that helps you toward your goals.

It is vital you are clear on this, if your appearance is not important, you will never be in great shape. It is as simple as that, you only work for something in your life which you feel is important. If you didn't think money was important you would not go to work, if you did not think sports were important you wouldn't watch them.

How you act is related to importance. There are some things in life that you have to do such as eat some food, drink water, sleep etc but the majority of our other behaviours are by choice. How you choose to spend that time is based on the importance you place upon it. The person who goes to the gym five times a week thinks it is important to be in shape and thinks going to the gym is an important element of this process. The person who rushes home after work to pick the kids up early from their child minder thinks it is important to spend time with their children. Your behaviours show the world what you think is important.

Everyone in great shape thinks it is important to look good and do the things that allows you to look good. It is as simple as that, it is the bottom line. Either accept it and incorporate it into your personality or spend your time going round in circles watching tiny hurdle after tiny hurdle trip you up.

When you believe something is important then behaviour change can happen very quickly. Have you ever heard of a woman who has struggled to give up drinking and cigarettes for years? Then one day she finds out she is pregnant and in the blink of an eye never touches a drop of alcohol or a cigarette for the nine months. Nothing had changed except importance. The cigarettes and drink still gave the same taste, same chemicals to the body, they were still as pointless an activity as they were before but the now pregnant lady has a goal on which she has placed a higher importance in this behavioural area and it is enough to create instant behavioural change.

If no one had told the woman about the devastating effects smoking and alcohol can have on a baby then why would she have changed her behaviour? The answer is she would not have changed.

What you need to do is to make being in great shape important. From this day forth you need to understand that being in amazing shape is something you should not just desire a little, but should crave. You must know that it is very important, that you deserve success and prioritise your behaviours to reflect this.

You can tell when someone truly thinks being in shape is important because they make things happen. The excuses are nonexistent and things somehow get done against all the odds. As their goal is important, it is involved in all their planning processes. Most people who pretend they take health and fitness seriously like to think of the necessary behaviours as an afterthought. They plan their day with work, kids and social events first then think about exercise as an afterthought. They shoot off to work in a panic under some false illusion that the company will fall apart if they are not there early and leave late while of course taking no breaks.

People in great shape plan the day ahead with full acceptance of how they need to contribute to their health and fitness goals. They do this because it is truly important to them. They get it done. People in amazing shape do not hide, the result is judged on how you look, not on how much you tried or how hard your life is. It is on how great you look on that beach, on holiday, in the biggest social gathering of the year. There is no hiding place. If getting in shape is important to you then start acting like it is.

One of the most frequent comments I hear is "yes, getting in shape is so important to me but I am just so...... (Insert excuse here)". I have had the pleasure of working with many people from almost every background and varying levels of 'success' in life. I have seen almost every personal situation with work, family, business allow for results.

The only real difference I found in terms of circumstances was how the person viewed them. I have worked with identical business owners working 70 hours a week. One complained life was too hectic, he never found time to prepare food or exercise. The other found the time to get to the gym, if he had a busy week where exercising was literally impossible he would make sure his eating was 100% on the money. Same situation, different result! The first businessman is still overweight many years on and second man is still in great shape. The only difference between these two was the value placed on success. One thought it was achievable alongside his other goals while the other spouted so many excuses he never even looked at potential solutions. Either way, the result stands, they can each look in the mirror to see.

Giving your goals equal priority to each other -

The amazing thing about health, fitness and getting in shape is it does not take as much time as people think. The key is not the time commitment it needs but it is the priority you must give it to sit alongside other goals. It is a fallacy that going to the gym needs to take more than 20 minutes if you are on a tight schedule, same with food, it doesn't take much more time to eat healthily than to eat rubbish. It just takes some priority at the beginning to allow it into your planning.

I have seen people attain success under almost every circumstance. New mothers jog with their prams, businessmen train before work, mother's of 6 children ensure they eat perfectly whatever the kids are up to, busy business executives only use hotels with the right food options, stressed employees negotiate flexitime to go to the gym at lunch time, 9-5 office workers who are also in a band find time to get to the gym and take food to their gigs. The situation is irrelevant, what you need to be successful is to label your health and fitness goal as equally important as your other goals. When I say label as equally important I mean just that. It does not need to come at the expense of other goals in your life.

You can be in amazing shape and have a good job, you can have a great family and be in amazing shape. There is no need for exclusivity. You do not need to prioritize one goal over another, your job does not need to be more important than your body or vice versa. This is because you are discussing independent variables.

How healthy you are is important in the areas of health, how rich you are is important in the area of money. Try buying a car with your good health or conversely try eating your money to get into great shape and be in good health. This analogy seems stupid but that is exactly what people do each day when they prioritize one goal over the other.

All you need to do is follow what every person in amazing shape does, prioritize their goal of being in great shape to be up there with other life goals, no higher and no lower but just on a equal scale.

It is common to see “life” easily overtake your goals. For example, the start of a new romantic relationship signals the death toll for your exercise and nutrition routines. The moment the relationship finishes the health and fitness efforts are stepped back up. People in amazing shape do not let their relationships compromise their efforts or desires to achieve their dream body. This is because they have equal priority in their minds.

If you spend fifty hours a week working it is hard to convince me you couldn’t find 2 hours to get three gym visits done. If you are working fifty hours a week it is absolutely essential to find 15 minutes a day to think and prepare the food that you will eat for the next day. Notice I am not saying give up work, become a full time gym addict, I am saying step up and stop whinging and find some balance in these two equally important goals. At the same time understand that your health goals impact on every other goal you have in your life. When your health and fitness are going well you are a better parent, better friend, more productive, more efficient and make better decisions. This benefits all aspects of your life.

Inspiration versus desperation -

One of the ways to ensure your goal is both important to you and also obtains equal priority is to ensure that it is inspirational. The majority of weight loss goals come out of total desperation rather than inspiration.

Desperation is the opposite of being inspired. When you are feeling inspiration it is aligning itself with the third tier of happiness, fulfilment. When you are desperate you will likely seek out false pleasure sources for your happiness to counter balance the emotions which come from feeling desperate. These simple pleasures usually come in the form of junk food or self abusive behaviour such as getting drunk. When acting out of inspiration there are no alternative behaviours because it is what you want to be doing. You are not working towards a goal you are part of an inspiring process. It is exactly what you want to do!

Desperation goals in regards to your weight are fundamentally flawed. They are based on the false premise that "I will be different when I achieve my goal". As discussed previously this occurs when you think must achieve your goal weight to feel a certain way. You are relying on achieving your goal to take the pain away. No wonder you are desperate! No-one wants to live that way.

The feelings of desperation are exacerbated if you do not progress towards your goals because this means you cannot remove the pain. However, this same pain has now been magnified by your ever so busy brain to be ten times worse than it ever was at the beginning of this process.

Even when you do start making progress it can still make you feel desperate because you may find that despite your progress it is not changing the pain you want to get rid of. This makes you panic so you think the pain must disappear if you lose more fat. If only you could get there faster.

Acting out of inspiration refers to how you are not trying to achieve a mystical goal in the distance to avoid pain but that you are doing the behaviours you want to be doing right here and now. This is because they inspire you. This style of thinking is less about the result and more about the process. It makes you feel alive and happy. People in great shape would act the way they do whether they were looking amazing like they do now or if they were out of shape.

This is because they are inspired by the process and pursuit of their goals, not solely focused on the end results. It appears easy for them to get where they want to be because they have done it through a natural desire to engage in the activities that bring success. People in great shape get an amazing buzz from doing the right things, while people who desperately chase their goal hold a great deal of resentment to the fact they are forced to eat 'good' foods just because they 'have' to achieve their goal. This is accentuated if you feel you have to achieve your goals to be happy, attractive, rich, proud, worthy or any other false attachment you have placed on succeeding.

You may be wondering how you gain inspiration to lose weight instead of feeling desperation. Inspiration comes from clearing your mind of the influences from family, friends, work colleagues etc who try to tell you how hard it is to do many of the tasks that a person in great shape finds inspiring. The general population (who are mostly all out of shape) view almost everything as a chore. If you are not careful you may just convince yourself that their poor opinions are actually fact. You need to tune into your body and mind to notice what feelings really excite you.

You will find that true inspiration and happiness in the form of satisfaction and fulfilment comes from doing the tasks that will help your body get into shape. You get an amazing buzz just after an exercise session. You do not after a night of drinking or stuffing yourself with junk foods. There is a great feeling of excitement when you try and add a new food to your diet which is full of goodness for your body, this lasts much longer and feels so much more aligned with the true you compared to sneaking a chocolate bar after dinner.

The activities that aid your body will truly give you a sense of satisfaction and fulfilment. People in amazing shape have discovered the inspiration within these activities. For you to tune into the inspiration you simply need to clear your mind and listen for these feelings. This is how you develop inspiration. Most of the common pleasure activities such as eating and drinking provide a small amount of temporary pleasure before going on to make you feel worse. If you tune into your own energy you will find these behaviours are not even close to the feelings you get from activities that help your body. Sometimes you must think outside of the box to find inspiration. For example, if you told me I had to run for twenty minutes on the treadmill I would hate it and never do it. If you said I had to do twenty minutes running outside I could just about grin and bear it. However, if you said I could do sprinting on the athletics track I would be ecstatic. It is all running to the outsider but a massive difference to the exerciser.

The problem with modern day life is that we have almost all forgotten what this inspired feeling is like. It has been sucked out of us by negative people, crushed by society, dampened by watching too much TV and so forth. You can see this in the way children have changed. In years gone by they would enjoy being inspired by going out to play with their friends. Kids of today miss out on this feeling from being stuck at home watching TV or on their computers. Playing games whilst out and about is an enjoyment that comes from within. Watching TV is hoping that an external object will bring you joy. The real crime is not only that our kids are forgetting / never learning what that feeling is but also that almost all of us adults have forgotten it too.

Benefits of being in amazing shape

Most people have never been in sensational shape and they do not know what life is like when you are. If you are in truly amazing shape (all four aspects – looks, fitness, health and mind) you are living with a freedom you have never had before. The mind is clear from worry, negative self talk or fears about what to wear, what people will think at social functions or what will happen during the summer holidays.

When you are in amazing shape you have a level of belief and self confidence that you never had before. You understand you are a good person and you are better able to both give out love and receive it from the world around you. You have the confidence to try and do things you always wanted.

When you are feeling wonderful you have an added spring in your step. A level of energy that sweeps you along to do things that you never thought were possible or would even have contemplated in years gone by. To wake up in the morning free from aches and pains while feeling good is an experience money cannot buy.

Perhaps the best benefit of being in amazing shape is your ability to help others. You can only ever pull people up to your level in life and not push them up from below. When you are operating at a higher level you are better able to help other people. The transformation that happens when you create your dream body carries over into every single area of your life from relationships to work to personal peace of mind.

It must be remembered that the benefits of being in shape come as a result of the journey over the actual results themselves. Becoming someone in amazing shape overnight will not bring with it the benefits if you have not changed your mindset too. As mentioned, very often you will have to first change mentally to induce the physical changes rather than the other way round. Start doing any activities today that make you feel happy, confident, attractive or free. The more you experience these feelings the quicker the process of transformation can occur.

BEHAVIOUR CHANGE EXERCISES

Awareness –

Write down a version of your goal that is purely inspirational. This means something you are bursting with excitement to do. It should fill you with joy just thinking about it. Your goal could inspire you in many areas of your life including – relationships, love, family, sex, recognition, friends, wealth, freedom.

With this inspirational goal in mind start making a note of other people who are in amazing shape yet also lead similar lives to yours, e.g. also have 3 children, work 50 hours a week etc.

Questioning –

What would you need to do to give your health and fitness goals equal priority to your other goals in life? How can you find inspiration in your health and fitness behaviours?

Intention –

Decide to be inspired by your goals and recognise that they are important enough to sit alongside

PRINCIPLE 3 – COMMIT TO YOUR GOALS THROUGH THE POWER OF ACTION

In the real world your results are achieved by actions. How you look depends on how much of the right foods you eat, how much of the wrong foods you avoid, how often you exercise etc. It is a game of actions and people in amazing shape take more action than people in awful shape.

Commitment

The word commitment brings up various pictures and images for different people. The usual view of commitment is stereotyped by the strict fitness freak versus the junk food eating 'slob'. The 'don't give a damn' out of shape person is not really whom I am talking about. They have no apparent desire to be in shape. A lack of commitment refers to a lack of action towards your goals. If you have no goals, you cannot show low commitment.

Actual low commitment is when you want to get in shape but never get the necessary actions done. Most people do not show low commitment. Almost everyone I have met has enough commitment, however almost all apply it in the wrong areas which gives the appearance they lack commitment.

Showing commitment in the wrong areas is analogous to driving a car at top speed in the wrong direction. You are going fast but you are not getting any closer to where you want to go. Commitment is usually seen as the ability to endure long hours, repeated failures, to get up when you have been knocked down, never quitting, depriving yourself etc. This is not my view. True commitment is doing the actions you need to do. This is made up equally of 'intelligent decisions' as it would be of 'will power and dedication'.

People in amazing shape do more of the right actions than people in worse shape. That does not mean they spend more time thinking, obsessing or worrying about their weight. They simply do more of the correct actions. For example, one person may spend hours worrying about what to eat, if they have their meal right, only to end up eating a poor meal for their body. A second person may spend five minutes planning a meal they know is 100% right for them. In terms of effort the first person clearly wins, in terms of commitment (doing the right actions) the second wins by a long way. Guess which one will be in great shape?

This is where we get it all wrong - effort and commitment are two completely different facets. We judge our commitment levels on the effort scale. This is an awful idea, because effort does not guarantee success and very often it is inversely related to it. The less efficient your health and fitness strategies, the harder you must try to get results. The difference between effort and commitment is that effort lets you off the hook by dropping your accountability for results. It allows you to say to yourself "well, I have put in this effort so I deserve this reward". It negates efficiency and decision making. The real world is based on results, would you congratulate your taxi driver if he had just driven an hour in the wrong direction? Why treat your body any differently?

Most people who are out of shape are putting effort in the wrong areas. We all love to focus on the areas we are strong at while avoiding the areas that prove more difficult. You think, "If I go to the gym five times this week I can eat a load of chocolate every night". This is a classic example of too much effort in the face of wrongly applied commitment. If the chocolate is what is causing you to be fat, then your commitment is measured by your actions of how much chocolate you do not eat, nothing else. However, we avoid this because it is easier to exercise than give up chocolate as no one has taught you how to change your behaviour.

In this example, true commitment is how much you address this issue. It is about how you learn about techniques to remove nutritional based food cravings and breaking emotional connections to food (chocolate). It is your commitment (actions) to break your chocolate addiction in which you should be judged and not by how many times you go to the gym. The latter makes you feel better because you can justify your efforts but ultimately it keeps you stuck because you are celebrating going in the wrong direction. You are avoiding a behaviour that is crucial to results.

You need to decide exactly what you need to be measuring commitment by, how do you measure commitment currently? When you find you have changed your approach to measuring commitment by judging the actions directly influencing results you will see a massive change in your fortunes. The only problem is these areas are more than likely going to be your weak points.

My definition of commitment also involves the aspects of intelligence and decision making, where intelligence is not to do with academic ability but rather the ability to make the right choices. This is based more on your intuition and then subsequent commitment to listen to that voice. For example, you may know that certain foods are not working for your body but choosing to act on that voice and eliminate them takes a commitment on your part as they could just be your current favourite foods.

True commitment often does not lead you to the most obvious decision, simply the right one. It may take the form of you greatly reducing your exercise when your body is over trained, despite this coming in the face of your fear of getting fat. It could mean increasing your carbohydrate intake after years of eating low carbs, or vice versa, all against a backdrop of fear that you may get out of shape. That is true commitment, taking the right decision in spite of current feelings. People in amazing shape make these decisions, they show true commitment.

Wanting versus resenting

One of the big blocks to commitment through action is resentment. It seems almost human nature that when someone orders you to do something you push back against them. The resistance is usually not against the request itself but it is against the mere fact you are being told to do something.

Most of us can remember times when we have wanted to do something but found one or more people suggest in an overly aggressive way that you should do it as well and then all of a sudden you decide against it. When your parents are involved this is even more common. It stems from years of being told what to do. In response, you simply take the opposite stance and point of view whether this is best for you or not and even if it is against something you actually want to do. You may feel resentment whenever someone says tidy your room, go to the shops, don't eat that, you need to lose weight etc.

This is very significant to losing body fat and getting into shape because many people in poor shape are resenting the fact they have to lose fat, they resent the fact they have to stop eating certain foods, they resent the fact they need to exercise, they resent almost everything to do with getting into shape. Such feelings are associated with comments like "Why do I have to ____" "It is not fair I cannot eat ______", "how come other people can do ___ but I cannot?"

The opposite of resentment is wanting, inspiration and desire. You should aim to want to do something because it inspires you and fills you full of excitement and energy. People in amazing shape do not resent exercising - they want to do it. They do not resent eating the right foods and reducing the wrong ones because they want to do it. They understand the same actions that allow them be in great shape also make them feel good. Life seems easier for these people because they are not battling resentment towards these behaviours. They are choosing to do them.

Feelings of deprivation are magnified by resentment. Resentment is linked to choice, apparent choice. If you have chosen to do the action because you want to do it (not because you have to do it) then you will not feel any resentment towards it. When you feel you have to do something you will feel a large emotional push in the opposite direction. This push tricks your mind into a dialogue such as "I have to give up bread because I have to be thin....But I really want bread, it is so unfair I cannot have bread, I resent the fact I cannot have bread....I feel so deprived, I can see my friends eating it and enjoying it....this is so unfair...I so want some bread"

This incessant dialogue in the mind is producing an endless battle. This is one of the reasons the nutrition strategies that allow you to eat what you want can prove effective. They work by banishing resentment from the mind so that you are free to choose what you want, which for many people is the exact foods they were trying to eat previously but couldn't stick to while battling their own resentment.

The way around resentment is open and free choice. It cannot live in the face of this. For this to happen you must drop the notion of being allowed to act a certain way. Understand you can act however you want but you are choosing to do everything to achieve your goal and that ultimately you want to attain this goal, you do not have to achieve it.

When to commit to success

At some point in your life you will need to commit towards and succeed in achieving your health and fitness goals. Either you will achieve them at some point in your life or you will go through life having never achieved them. In general, the longer you wait to achieve your goals the harder it becomes. Once you have succeeded, maintaining results is easier than the process of achieving them. This principle is the same in any endeavour.

To build a business you must devote a portion of your life to growing it. If you have used the right structure in your business then it will become self sustaining after a while and require much less effort to maintain long term. Our retirement model is based on this same premise. You earn money early in your life through effort so you can create a passive income source, e.g. pension etc when you are older and thus do not have to work unless you choose to.

The body requires you to put in some effort to get it to the level that it needs to be and then maintaining it is much easier. The time it takes to get there is very much dependent on what your body has done so far and its capabilities to adapt. In general, the younger you are the easier it is to fix. The older you are the more time that has passed in which the body can go wrong. This is from your actions as well as the natural cumulative effects of ageing. In regards to achieving your goal, you need to ask yourself a few questions:

Will I ever achieve my goal?
When will I achieve it?
What is stopping me achieving it?

The answer to first question should be a 100% yes! If is anything along the lines of "maybe", "it would be nice", "hopefully" then you need to decide it is ok to do the behaviours to get in shape even if you are not successful. Most people only take action when they believe they will be successful. Without the belief they only ever go half heartedly and do not show the necessary commitment (actions) needed for success. People in amazing shape go after their goals with all guns blazing. They do not do things half heartedly. You must do the same with or without the belief that you will be successful.

Alternatively, if you do not have any real plans on achieving your goal, then save yourself the bother and change your goal to something that you do really intend to achieve. Often we set goals that we do not truly want. We say we would like these goals because others want it or it seems the thing to do. The key to successful motivation and thus commitment is a genuine inspirational desire to want the goal.

When you have this you will understand that at some point in your life you are going to have to commit 100% to it. This means choosing to do every action possible to make it happen. You do not have to do this today, or next week. However, you must realise that at some point it has to happen. The switch in your head has to click and you step up to the plate and realise that you are doing this and no one, no thing or no excuse will let you be knocked off track. When you make the decision that the time is now every action you take comes out of choice and inspiration. Resentment and desperation is thrown from the ranks and no longer becomes an issue.

The best time to start this is always NOW. The longer you wait the further away the start date becomes and the more time you have to disrupt your body. There will always be another problem that prevents you starting, your life is always hectic so the best time to begin is pretty much always NOW.

Once you have committed, you can then work on the answers to what is stopping you achieving your goal. Please bear in mind your reason very often is not the real reason why you are not achieving your goals. This book should open your eyes to the real reasons and true commitment will allow you to be brave enough to follow through on the actions your body is asking for. Once you are committed you will of course be working on developing the subconscious programming to make all your behaviour automatic. At this point you will show commitment long term without even thinking about it. This is the recipe for long term results and joining the tiny percentage of the population who are in amazing shape.

BEHAVIOUR CHANGE EXERCISES

Awareness –

Write down the answers to the following questions:

What behaviours are you holding resentment towards having to do?

What areas are you putting in effort but not getting the actions done?

Questioning –

What is the cause of the resentment you are feeling towards the behaviours identified in the awareness section? How can you ensure you take more actions yet expend less effort?

Intention

Make a pact with yourself today to measure progress only by the number of right actions taken. While doing this, understand you choose to do all these behaviours and you do not have to do any behaviour. In fact, you do not even have to achieve your goal. It is all your choice.

Touch your hand on your heart and say out loud ten times:

"I take action Now! I measure progress by actions completed and choose to do the actions that bring success"

Planning –

Review the areas where you are putting in the most effort yet getting little done, e.g. avoiding bread at lunch, going to the gym before work. Create a plan where you can convert this effort into action. Note down what you need to do to change your behaviour in this situation. Often it is something very subtle, e.g. buying a lunch box, having a shorter exercise routine. Commit to success by taking action to resolve this block immediately, e.g. taking lunch to work to avoid having to have sandwiches, going to the gym for just twenty minutes.

Emotional management –

Remove the resentment you have to any individual behaviour you are rebelling against. Use

Emotional Freedom Technique (EFT) to achieve this. (See www.benwilsonuk.com for an EFT demonstration). Simply fill in the blanks and then tap the EFT points while saying the statement below. Repeat for all the behaviours you are showing resentment towards:

"Even though I resent __________ I deeply and completely accept myself and decide to do this behaviour out of choice"

e.g. "Even though I resent having to give up chocolate I deeply and completely accept myself and decide to do this behaviour out of choice"

PRINCIPLE 4 – USE EMOTIONAL OUTLETS THAT DO NOT INVOLVE FOOD OR DRINK

Whether you are in amazing shape or poor shape one thing which is certain is that you have emotions to battle against. The question is how do you handle them? People in amazing shape have equally as much negative emotion as those in poor shape. What they do differently however, is to use more emotional outlets that do not involve food or drink than their out of shape counterparts. The amount of emotional stress you are experiencing is outlined in figure 8:

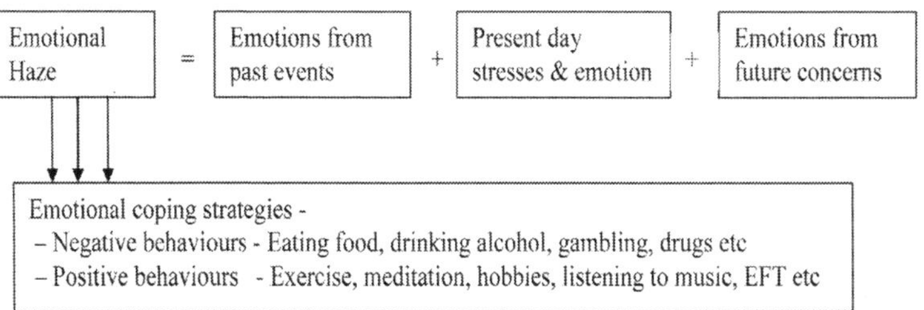

Figure 8 – Influences on your emotional stress

The ability to handle emotions is one of the most important of all strategies to be in amazing shape. This is because it will free you from being tied to food and drink for support and allow you to choose the right foods. If you want to know how you are wired for coping at the moment then just look at your current behaviours, especially in times of increased emotional stress.

It is impossible to have a discussion on emotional eating unless you are fully aware of the different types of hunger. Most people are better at coping with their emotions than they give themselves credit for but the problem is that most people are very bad at controlling the different types of hunger. Therefore, nutritional based cravings become mislabelled as emotional desires for food.

The six types of hunger

Most people think hunger is just hunger but this is not the case. There are in fact six types of hunger. It is vital you understand what these are otherwise you will find yourself addressing emotional issues when you should be addressing nutritional ones and vice versa. In my experience the nutritional reasons account for way over 50% of most peoples' cravings and in some cases 100%. This means that you are blaming yourself for being weak willed and a bad person when the truth is you are simply miscalculating what you should eat. Let me explain more about each of the types of hunger:

Normal hunger –

Normal hunger is a natural and calm desire for food. The hunger builds gradually and evenly. It can usually be battled against fairly well until it rises to a high level. This natural feeling should be listened to. This hunger will always be present throughout your life and should be satisfied when it arises. When this is the only type of hunger you experience in your life you will feel calm, controlled and have an easy relationship with food.

Water hunger –

A thirst for water is almost indistinguishable from a normal hunger feeling. It usually grows gradually and evenly. It will be like normal hunger in that it is a fairly calm request on the body and you can easily manage it. However, if you always eat food instead of drinking you may find yourself continually eating and not understanding why. A water hunger may often occur without you actually feeling thirsty. A water hunger is easily countered by drinking water regularly throughout the day.

Cell energy hunger –

A cell energy hunger is one of the most common causes of hunger and perhaps the biggest reason people wrongly blame their eating on emotions. A cell energy hunger comes when you eat a meal with the incorrect ratio of Protein: Carbohydrates: Fat for your body. When this happens you will get a hunger feeling, often in the form of a sugar craving, anywhere from 15 minutes up to 3 hours after eating. This is usually the reason that you can find yourself hungry fairly soon after having a meal despite the fact you "should" be full.

The way to counter this is to eat each meal with the correct ratio of Protein: carbohydrates: Fat for your body. This can be found out through experimentation and using food reaction forms.

Blood sugar hunger –

This is a powerful hunger. When your blood sugar levels drop below a certain value your hormone system kicks in to regulate your metabolism. This puts an unwelcome stress on your body long term and in the short term produces some very strong food cravings and hunger. The onset can be fast. When certain values are hit in your blood glucose levels you will be hungry and this can become a strong sugar craving. A large percentage of the population suffer low blood sugar throughout the day.

Low blood sugar problems can be resolved in the short term by eating regularly and ensuring you are eating in accordance to your ideal ratio of protein to carbohydrates to fat. However, blood sugar metabolism is a sign of many different factors and processes. Therefore, long term resolution comes from addressing your body's overall functioning and health.

Deficiencies hunger –

This refers to a craving or hunger due to a deficiency within the body. There are different possible underlying causes to this. Some experts say it is due to neurotransmitter imbalances, others low glycogen levels in the liver, deficiencies in certain vitamins / minerals or issues of food reward/ palatability. Regardless of the source a deficiency hunger operates in the background as a sort of uneasy feeling. The hunger neither comes nor goes, it is just there affecting you and drawing you into the food. This is almost always mistakenly viewed as an emotional hunger.

Emotional hunger –

True emotional hunger has nothing to do with nutritional cravings. An emotional craving has a very fast onset, often instantaneously. You see a picture of a chocolate bar in a magazine and all of a sudden you are craving it, you receive a phone call that makes you angry and immediately you are snacking on some biscuits. Maybe you speak to someone about money and straightaway you are having a cake. It could be you meet someone who reminds you of a person from your past and you descend into a night of drinking. The emotional cause of your poor eating may be obvious, e.g. just broke up with partner, or you may be oblivious if deep within the subconscious. The general lack of happiness in your life is also a contributing factor for emotional eating, e.g. deriving pleasure from eating a certain food to make up for a lack of other things in your life which make you happy.

The interplay of the different hungers –

It is when you experience more than one hunger simultaneously that most people crack and end up eating junk. The most common reason being an emotional hunger in combination with one of the other nutritional based hungers. It is difficult to avoid eating poorly when suffering more than one type of hunger, yet plenty of people go on day after day in this state.

Fear of hunger

Many people hold a fear of hunger which is often a cause in itself for desperation eating. At the first sign of any hunger, which may be a natural and a normal hunger feeling you panic and eat ASAP with whatever is within grabbing distance. This same fear also takes holds when you know you cannot eat for a few hours. You therefore eat much more than you need to eat to ensure you make it through to the next meal.

As a society the view to hunger has changed in recent years. In years gone by it was common to have to wait until lunch or dinner time to eat your food. In this modern day we are encouraged (and able) to eat at the first signs of hunger whatever time it is and however close you are to your next meal. There is a feeling that experiencing a slight bit of hunger and having to wait an hour for dinner could be likened to suffering starvation amidst a famine. In years gone by this was not the case. You would be told by your parents that dinner would be ready in an hour and you would have to grin and bear it. You were given a set amount of food to take to school or work and that was your lot.

While experiencing hunger is not ideal because it is a sign from your body that it wants something, it is also not a reason to panic and eat the first bit of junk food in sight. When you follow the right plan your hunger is controlled and you suffer few cravings. Follow the wrong nutritional plan and the opposite occurs. Therefore let hunger be a sign to address your nutritional plan until it is controlled and resolved rather than the green light to eat everything in sight.

I still meet people day in day out who are trying to starve themselves thin. This method never allows you to be in amazing shape as it goes against your biochemistry and is totally unnecessary. Strong hunger is a request from your body. It means you need to change your nutrition plan. It is not something to fight against.

Strategies for controlling your emotions

The way you react to your emotions is neither right nor wrong, it is just that certain coping strategies will aid your body and others will ruin it. Most people eat junk food or drink to handle their emotions. If you want to look amazing it is necessary to ensure you use enough positive strategies to raise your behaviour level above the threshold for results. When reviewing your current strategies I suggest you do not berate yourself up for anything you currently do. It is simply the best coping strategy that you have come up with so far, nothing more, nothing less. It may be disastrous for your body but rather than moping about the past, let's look at the way forward.

If you were experiencing no emotional stress you would have no reason to use your coping strategies. Likewise, if your only response to excessive emotions was eating perfectly and exercising at the correct level you would not need to worry about your emotions neither.

The best approach for handling your emotions is to find coping methods that do not involve food or drink and reduce your emotions below the level that requires you to use such methods to cope. The coping techniques used are very important because everyone will have ups and downs in emotions. To ensure success look to reduce your emotions from the past, present and future concerns so that you have a large reserve to handle even the most stressful of emotional events that come up within your life.

Overview of negative emotional coping behaviours

The negative behaviours used in an attempt to control the emotions include some that ruin the body and others which may have negative effects on other areas of your life. Some of the most common include:

Using food or drink –

This is usually the major one for almost everyone and definitely for people who are out of shape. When using food to control your emotional stress most of us fall into a pattern of choosing just one or two foods. These favourite foods become an emotional prop.

Food has a very limited impact on your emotions, worse still, poor food choices upset your biochemistry which makes you less able to handle emotions. The reason people grab for food is that it is readily available and because it masks and distracts your mind for a short period of time. Food or drink does not provide any substantial form of happiness nor does it reduce excess emotions. This means you are simply distracting the mind but you are still left in the same situation. The result will be you need to repeat the behaviour again just a few minutes to hours later. If the emotional stimulus has gone then things will improve but otherwise the food will be there, calling.

Some people allow the emotions to build then have a huge binge on food. This appeases the mind up to a point but it is only a matter of time before you repeat the process. It could be that you binge on Saturday and that tides you over to the next weekend. This is a form of the willpower method. If I have a big intake now, I can last it out until to the next weekend. The problem is you are still at the mercy of emotions. If it is a tough week you may gorge on food on a Thursday night. If it was a real tough week you gorge every night and still it has no effect. Though food can provide some pleasure (true or false pleasure) people mostly use it as a distraction to try to mask their emotions.

Smoking –

Smoking is another negative coping behaviour with the added issue of ruining your lungs and cardiovascular system. Smokers get a bad press to say the least and I certainly do not condone the behaviour but you could make an argument that it is worse to eat junk food than it is to smoke. The Japanese top the life expectancy charts[6] yet the country consumes the third most cigarettes in the world[7]. You should not be rushing off to take up smoking because once the smoking becomes less effective on your emotions (as it does) you will start eating junk foods as well. Smoking fails you just like food because it does not reduce your emotions!

Obsessive and addictive behaviours – over exercising, too much work, internet addiction, TV, gambling, sex

There are numerous other addictions and obsessive behaviours we may substitute for eating and drinking. If these do not involve food or drink then you can almost guarantee that they are going to be more helpful for your body shape than the previous methods. However, in my opinion the mind should feel as good as the body looks to be someone truly in amazing shape. Any addiction undermines how good we feel.

There is a fine line between a natural passion or joy and an addiction. In general, an addiction is something you cannot give up at that level even if you wanted to, while a positive love for it is something we choose to do and can stop if needed. It is a fine line. Exercise, sex, surfing the internet, TV, gambling etc can all prove legitimate methods for dissipating emotions. They are good in that they do not involve food and drink but if used in a way that they become an unhealthy obsession then it can spell trouble.

This is what I often see with people who are training at the gym twice a day. They are doing it out of fear of getting fat. Unbeknown to them this same activity is often contributing to them having trouble losing fat. This is a very different scenario to an athlete who is inspired to win a competition who is training twice a day. They are able to and do take time off to ensure the body recovers. The obsessed exerciser only stops when the body gives up and they are ill in bed

The reasons all these methods fail when dealing with emotions is that they bring with them negative consequences and are aimed at trying to divert attention away from the stress rather than trying to address the emotions experienced head on.

Overview of positive strategies to control your emotional stress

The most effective way to handle emotions is to use activities that do not harm the body and not only distract your mind from the emotions but reduce the actual emotions you are experiencing. This is the way to achieve effortless results long term. I will run through the major possible methods at your disposal but the list is only limited by your imagination.

Emotional reduction strategies –

There are numerous strategies to reduce negative emotions. These work in various ways but all serve to neutralise the emotion you are experiencing. This means you no longer feel sad, guilty, angry etc when you think about the issue that was previously upsetting you. This is the opposite of trying to mask your emotions with food.

There are various techniques you can use. The list includes Emotional Freedom Technique (EFT), Thought Field Therapy (TFT), Neuro Linguistic Programming (NLP), Psych-K, Integral Eye Movement Therapy (IEMT), Cognitive Behaviour Therapy (CBT) amongst many other techniques. There are also numerous therapist based counselling techniques. Different techniques have their merits and the ultimate test is what works for you.

To this there are also approaches that look more into the nature of thought and how we function. These include mindfulness and the "3 Principles Movement" as well as other philosophical or spiritual teachings

My personal favourites are Emotional Freedom Technique (EFT) which you have already encountered in the behaviour change exercises set out previously and the 3 Principles. The former is an easy to use tool in the moment while the latter allows you to change your whole relationship to thought and stress.

I also like the other techniques too. You may find different strategies work better for you than the above. A key element though is ability to use it regularly, on your own and in a way that reduces your stress and negative emotions. The more of these skills you learn and the higher your level of mastery the more in control of your mind-body you will become.

Meditation, visualization, emotional and spiritual healing –

These techniques are similar in their form as they involve spending a few minutes to quieten the mind and thus allowing you to relax. This is a good strategy and can be massively beneficially to your mindset. A daily meditation can do wonders.

A point to note on meditations / healing is that they often have a different effect to the emotional reduction strategies listed previously. Experiment with these techniques to see what works best for you but often the best policy is to combine both types of approach.

Hobbies –

These days it is becoming rarer and rarer to find people with hobbies. This is such a shame and is no surprise that it is yet another correlation with our increasing waist lines. Hobbies are awesome. They are something you enjoy, you choose to do and they usually fill you with inspiration, which aligns itself with the higher levels of happiness.

Hobbies come in all shapes and sizes but recently they have become replaced with mindless TV watching. When you are engaged in your hobby you have much better things to do than eat or worry about your problems in your life because you are concentrating on something and losing yourself in your passion.

There are no rights or wrongs to hobbies. A hobby is simply something you really enjoy doing. It could be going to a dance class, riding horses, playing sports, playing a musical instrument, chess, fishing, gardening, languages, ice skating, drawing, painting, writing, sewing, knitting, walking, swimming, making models, acting, singing, yoga, meditation, pets and many more.

Everyone should have a few hobbies. A hobby should be something that inspires you but at the same time does not have too much emotional involvement in terms of your ego.

Activities without ego appeal to inspiration. When you start confusing your hobby for something that determines yourself worth (ego) then it becomes a little serious. You think, "I must make this picture I am painting good otherwise I will be a bad artist and then that means I am a bad person which means........" all of a sudden your hobby is now contributing to your emotions. When doing your hobby you should just do it for the love of it. When this happens you will find yourself inspired and inspiration reduces your negative emotions.

Reading the right books –

Reading is a great method for coping with your excessive emotions. Look to find books that inspire you and try to avoid books that depress, bore or link to negative events from your past. The more inspirational the book, the greater its effect on allowing you to handle any excess emotions without food.

If the bulk of your emotions stem from your present tense evaluation of life then it is very important for you to read personal development books that can aid in changing your emotions. Books work differently to TV because they engage the mind. So if you are feeling stressed open up your favourite book.

Exercise –

Using exercise as way to cope with your excess emotions is very powerful. It is a win-win situation. Doing it not only stops you eating junk food but it also accelerates progress towards your goals. The key for making exercise a strategy for handling your emotions is that it needs to be enjoyable.

For this to happen you must find the form of exercise that suits you best. It could be that you find an exercise class or a running club inspiring. Alternatively, it could be the gym or training alone outside is more motivating to you. The key is discovering what you like the most currently and then adjusting over time as your preferences change.

If you are the kind of person who does not have a clue how to exercise, then your first step is learning how to both do it and enjoy it. Until you know what you are doing and feel comfortable doing it then exercise can never become an emotional management technique.

Find a way to make exercise enjoyable for you. I have not met many people who do not enjoy exercise when they are taught it correctly. The key is learning to enjoy it. Sadly, way too many people have negative associations of exercise from the past.

When you enjoy exercise you will find yourself naturally thinking, "What a tough day, I am going to do some training". Almost every person in amazing shape has developed exercise as their primary way to handle emotions.

Helping people –

When you help people it gives you great feelings of satisfaction, fulfilment and enlightenment. It is a powerful way to help yourself emotionally and great for the other person too. Helping others is a gift you give out. It could be in a small way or through a larger favour. The key for you to receive the benefits of helping is to do it unconditionally. All too often when you help someone it is in exchange for something at a later date. This takes away the inspiration you receive from it. Look to give help to other people but for no other reason than to enjoy the experience of giving.

Ways to give and help people could include visiting a friend in need, helping a neighbour, volunteering a few hours a week for a good cause, helping your children with their projects, fundraising, doing sponsored events or simply paying someone a genuine compliment. The more you help people unconditionally the better you feel and this will allow you to handle your emotional stress more easily.

Doing tasks that bring satisfaction or doing things that are fun –

Performing any task that produces great satisfaction is more worthwhile than using food and drink to try to curb your emotions. Often these things can be your hobbies but other times it can be regular household tasks. I love cleaning things up when the house is very messy. It brings a good sense of satisfaction. Infuriatingly for anyone who lives with me though is that I have very little interest in tidying anything before it gets into a state of disaster.

When it comes to doing things that are fun, the list is almost endless. It could be going to the cinema, a concert, sports match, museum, theatre, dancing in the house to music, playing with the dog, days out to the zoo, the park or anything else that does not involve food or drink. These are similar to hobbies but the difference is, a hobby is something you do regularly. You may only go to the theatre once a year and the cinema occasionally. If you are feeling a bit down or life is getting too much then go and do something you enjoy.

Listening to music

Music is one of the most soothing ways that you can ease away emotions. Playing your favourite songs or music that reminds you of good times is a powerful way of eclipsing any negative emotions felt. If you want to, then dance and sing along as well. Music opens a pathway to freedom and happiness like no other method can.

An iPod should be a must have tool for anyone wanting to get into shape. When you are feeling down you can release and energise your spirit with your favourite songs. Music can also be a good tool to evoke emotions which can be broken down using EFT or similar emotional reduction technique.

Planning the future

A powerful and immediate path to inspiration is planning a future event. Inspiration and hope are both at the same level. When you are planning future events, be this a holiday, new house, wedding, career, business, a hobby, children or one of many thousands of other possibilities it fills you with hope, excitement and inspiration. I suggest you buy a blank book to use as a planning book. This is a powerful way to feel good. Instead of eating food and feeling miserable you can instead open up your planning book and begin to detail possible future actions you would like to do and how to do it. Before you know it, you will be full of warmth and feel a renewed enthusiasm.

Other possibilities – TV, films, spending time with your partner, friends.

There are other ways to behave outside the ones above when you are feeling an excess of emotions and have the desire to eat or drink. Other strategies are watching TV or films. In this area you must be careful it does not descend into mindless and de-motivational TV watching just for the sake of it. Sex is another great way to spend time with your partner and is yet another method which is better than eating junk food. Ensure that any time spent with someone does not have a behavioural anchor that says you should both eat junk food when together. If it does, then break that anchor so you can just spend time without ruining your body.

BEHAVIOUR CHANGE EXERCISES

Awareness –

Identify the major emotional coping strategies you use at the moment. Try and distinguish when you would use each one and how this relates to a particular emotion. It can be difficult to think of all these now if you are not experiencing the emotion, so it may be necessary to complete as and when these emotions come up. Not every negative emotion will produce a bad behavioural response. It is about identifying which ones will and addressing these. Write down how you react when experiencing each of the emotions listed in the table below.

Angry	–
Worried / anxious / fearful	–
Sad / unhappy	–
Bored / at a loose end	–
Lonely	–
Frustrated	–
Overwhelmed / busy	–
Tired	–
Happy	–

When celebrating –
Other –

Questioning –

Why do you react with negative behaviours for some emotions but not to others? What would it take for you to use positive coping strategies for all these emotions?

Intention.

Commit to realising that using food to address emotional reasons is never the most effective strategy and does not help you at all. Touch your hand on your heart and say out loud ten times:

"Eating food for any emotional reason is pointless! I use other strategies to control my emotions"

Planning –

Using your answers from the awareness section. Identify possible non food or drink related coping strategies to be used instead of the negative ones you are using now. These must be in a ball park of being an emotional equivalent. For example, saying you will drink water when you crave a chocolate bar to relax is probably not an emotional equivalent, however, listening to your favourite relaxing piece of music in the bath may well be.

Emotional management –

As well as using your equivalent behaviour technique the simultaneous use of emotional anchors to provide good feelings can also be a powerful strategy.

Ensure you have developed your anchors to use as a coping strategy. We have already set up two main anchors so far, one for excitement, happiness and feeling good. The second was for motivation to achieve your goal.

The final anchor you should develop is one for relaxation. To do this touch your thumb and middle finger together on your left hand (this is a different finger to the anchor for happiness). Ideally put on a piece of music you find relaxing. Keeping your fingers together, close your eyes and think about the most peaceful moment of your life so far, a time where you felt calm and relaxed. Spend two minutes reliving this. While keeping your thumb and middle finger together spend another two minutes thinking about something in the future where you will really feel relaxed. This could be an upcoming holiday.

Whenever you find yourself stressed touch your left thumb and middle finger back together and you will be reminded of this soothing sense of peace. Like with all anchors you may need to repeat this exercise a few times until the anchor is strong enough to produce real world relaxation.

PRINCIPLE 5 - AVOID MAKING EXCUSES AND TAKE RESPONSIBILITY

When it comes to some of the main reasons certain people get results while others do not the issue of excuses is often near the top of the list. The subject of excuses and making it happen represents the bridge between knowledge and application.

In the world of getting results there are no excuses I am afraid. You can cite this reason or that, explain why you couldn't do this, or were forced to eat that, but you are either getting results or you are not.

When you walk into a room at a party or restaurant looking fantastic with your clothes fitting perfectly or stumble in trying to hide under as many layers as possible there are no excuses at this point. You will know exactly where you are physically. Other people may try to say you look good but you are not easily tricked.

Excuses may make you feel fine in the moment that they were made but come the day, you want to be looking and feeling your best, you will not be listening to excuses. You will instead be unhappy about the reality before you.

Accepting responsibility

The first place to start in the quest to eradicate excuses is to take responsibility for what is yours to control and disown responsibility of what is outside of your control. This is very important as a big difference between people who achieve their goals and those that do not is in knowing what they can control and when to leave it be.

Accepting responsibility is the opposite of excusing yourself and forces you to act against the perceived block. This is the initial step before action occurs. Remember action is the be all and end all of getting results. It is your actions that you do (or not do) that will change your physical appearance.

Most people choose not to accept responsibility for their actions because it is easier to do so. It gives you a get out clause and allows you to feel better about yourself, I couldn't do this because of some other reason, as opposed to I couldn't do this because I am ....a bad person, weak willed, a failure or whatever other false assumption you make about yourself.

Almost every overweight person I have met are too harsh on themselves. They rapidly jump to the wrong conclusion about their behaviours. The reason they live by excuses is because the alternative conclusion that they jump to is so harsh on themselves it is much easier and safer to live with the excuse. The lack of logical reasoning in this area is a big problem. For example, perhaps at lunch the overweight person had a bit of chocolate, they use the excuse they didn't have time to prepare lunch so it was all they could eat. If they didn't hold this excuse they might jump to the conclusion they are too weak willed to resist chocolate and that they are a bad person etc.

The reality could be they had low blood sugar, or it could be they just have too much stress in their life and no one has taught them a better method of handling it. Whatever the reason, if you accept responsibility for the action this opens the door for resolving the problem. If more people would accept their behaviours as a signal from the mind-body instead of casting judgement on themselves it would allow a large amount of excuses to be dropped and many problems to be solved.

What to accept and what not to accept responsibility for

You should be accepting responsibility for as many actions as possible. This includes what you eat in a regular day, exercise in a typical week, taking and preparing food to eat, controlling your emotional outlets, self development, how you act when in the company of other people and their influences upon you. These are all vital action areas and under your control. You should assume charge of these areas, remove excuses and search for solutions to each problem that comes up.

Accepting responsibility also means taking it upon yourself to find out the way to get results. It is not your trainer's, doctor's or nutritionist's role to sort your body out however much you pay them to help. They are there to provide information and it is your responsibility to choose who gives you that information to help. You must then put it into action. If this does not obtain the desired results then you will move on to the next stage of the plan. People in amazing shape are in control of their plan of action. People who are out of shape are passive and rely on others to take control.

You should not assume responsibility for results. This is the responsibility of the body. Assume total responsibility for your actions yes, but not for your results. There is a subtle difference. The body is an amazing physiological structure but it is not under your direct control and you cannot predict 100% of the time how it will act.

You can have a perfect week's eating and exercising yet not lose any fat. This could happen for three weeks running and then you drop a massive amount of fat in that fourth week. If you are taking hold of your actions you should be happy and celebrate your success in those first few weeks regardless of the results. With the right mindset you will of course be looking and checking to see if this is the right plan you are following but assuming this is correct, do not make demands about how the body reacts.

If you do you will be linking your efforts to results and this is something you cannot predict. When things do not go your way it will cause anger, annoyance and an eventual 'giving up' of the health and fitness way of life. A point to note is you cannot give up on a health and fitness way of life. By being alive you are automatically in the game and it will never go away. Either you decide to play it well or play it poorly. You just have to live with your choices.

As well as not making demands of your results based on what you believe 'should be enough' I would also make allowances for irregular events such as birthdays, celebrations etc. These one off's cannot really do too much damage unless you regularly have irregular events. This comes down to having a balance in your life and your health and fitness behaviours (See Principle Seven).

There will also be times in which you literally could not avoid doing something because the actual circumstances forced you into it. In these cases do not hold any negative feelings about what happened and instead think of a counter measure you can do when you are back in control of the situation to make up for it.

Using responsibility for results

Whenever you make an excuse about a behaviour that you should have done but didn't, you should stop and ask, why did I behave in this way? By being in ownership of the behaviour you can now analyse why it happened. This is different to 'knowing' why it happened and blaming it on that external influence or worse still casting judgements about yourself.

Personally I am not immune to eating junk food like everyone else as I experience emotions and I have various anchors to the past associated with food as well as being subjected to the continual brainwashing society provides us. However, when I do observe my eating go awry I look for the signal about why I am doing this. I use the assumption that I am a good person and I am trying my best so why I am doing this behaviour? By using this approach you will not make numerous excuses, you will not cast doomsday judgements about yourself and more importantly you will eventually get to the bottom of why you are doing it. If you are tempted to eat junk food then ask yourself these two questions:

Why do I want to do this?

What would I need in my life to not need to do this behaviour?

This will take you towards the real reasons you want to eat and allow you to identify if you are making up an excuse or if it is a genuine reason your eating is going awry or can't get to the gym etc. Often you will find that it is a tiny block that stops you. In this situation simply becoming aware of it will often be enough to resolve it.

The reality could be that you do not have time for an hour long gym session, therefore go for just twenty minutes. Maybe you forgot to bring your food to work, so buy a 'healthy' lunch on the way to work (while you are not hungry) for later. If a tiny block like the above cannot be resolved by a simple behaviour change (most can) then it is more than likely you are doing this behaviour because you want to at an emotional level.

In the times you are doing something because you actually want to, e.g. you want to eat that chocolate, get drunk etc then you should not beat yourself up but instead start looking at why you want to do this behaviour and how you can change it (if necessary). It is important to use rational thought to solve the problem rather than being a harsh critic and berating yourself for being the worst person on the planet like most people do.

All your behaviours and actions are done for a reason. Eating that cake is for a reason, getting drunk is for a reason, going to or not going to the gym is for a reason. Criticising yourself for these actions is not productive as it only makes you feel bad. Analysing why you did something is the first step in behaviour change (awareness).

Avoid excuses in your health and fitness behaviours –

For results to happen you need to cut out the excuses in all aspects of your behaviours towards health and fitness.

Become a detective and look at every behaviour, thought and feeling you possess because they all come from somewhere. I have lost count of how many overweight people tell me they have no motivation. That is their excuse why they have failed to get results.

If they accept responsibility of their thoughts and actions they can stop the excuses and judgements about themselves and begin to ask the more important questions, what is motivation and will power to me? What do I mean by not having it and most importantly how can I create will power?

If you are accepting responsibility for your behaviour and thus asking why am I doing what I do then you will eventually work it out. If you are laying the blame at being weak willed, you will never solve the problem and you will just feel bad about yourself.

Another key element for avoiding excuses is ensuring you are doing things because you want to do it. When this is the case you will not need to find an excuse to get out of doing that task because you are keen to do it. This for many people is the hardest element as it relates to finding inspiration in both achieving your goal but also in doing the tasks that will bring you success. If you can find inspiration and enjoyment in eating the right foods, exercising and discovering what gets you results then the battle is about won.

BEHAVIOUR CHANGE EXERCISES

Awareness –

For the next week, whenever you find yourself making an excuse in any aspect of your life flick yourself on your right ear. Do not do it too hard, but do remember each excuse is ruining your body so maybe the harder you do it the sooner you will get the message.

This game is often more effective if you and a friend do it so you can point out when the person needs to flick their own ears. If your ear gets sore you will soon be getting the message. To start, think of three excuses you have already made today and get going by repeating each one out loud and flicking your ear.

Questioning –

Look at the excuses that seem to come up in your life time after time. For each excuse / behaviour ask yourself these two questions:

Why do I want to do this behaviour? (Or why do I never do this behaviour?)

What would I need in my life to resolve this problem?

For example, why do I want to eat this chocolate? Why do I never go to the gym? What would I need in my life to never eat chocolate / always go to the gym?

Intentions –

Decide from today forwards to be responsible for parts of your world that you can control and accept the things that are not in your control. As a result, drop all excuses from today onwards. Touch your hand on your heart and say out loud ten times:

"I take full responsibility for my actions. I get things done by finding a way!"

Planning –

Using your answers from the questioning section above, devise a plan where you can provide everything you need to break the underlying reasons for your excuses. Look to implement these ASAP.

Emotional management –

Identify the negative emotions you have about yourself that underlie the reasons you need to make excuses. Do not be shy, write down what you think about yourself. For example you may write I am weak willed, I am a bad person, I have no discipline, I am lazy. These thoughts are in your mind so put them on paper.

Now write next to your answer the name of someone who is worse than you in this aspect and someone who is better than you. For example, if you are lazy, write down the name of someone who is even lazier than you and also someone who is less lazy. This will allow you to begin to see your problems differently and that you are not the only person in the world with this issue. Remember that it is ok to have this problem and that you are still a great person however how you act. Congratulate yourself for simply trying to improve yourself. It is better than what most people do.

PRINCIPLE 6 - TAKE AN INTEREST IN HOW TO GET INTO AMAZING SHAPE

Taking an interest in being in shape is vital to success. It is even more vital for success if you are currently not in the shape you want to be. When you look at the difference between people in great shape and those that are not then a significant difference is how much interest they take in the project of achieving the body they want.

People who look good have taken the time to learn how things work for them. People in awful shape have not. Instead of delving into the different aspects of achieving results they instead rely on generalised advice from questionable sources, e.g. magazines. For results you need to take an active interest in discovering the system that works for you.

Biochemical individuality

An important element when taking an interest in being in great shape is understanding biochemical individuality. This is the term used to describe how as humans we are all unique.

You will recall from section one that this means the foods and behaviours that work for your best friend, partner or family member may not work for you. So when I say take an interest in being in great shape, I really mean, take an interest in discovering what strategies work for you (discover how individual your own biochemistry is). I have spent many years doing this for myself personally and on behalf of many clients. It never fails to amaze me the difference between any two people and the way certain factors affect one person but not the other. To get results you must find out what works for you.

Biochemical individuality exists because humans, like all animals, are subject to the influences of natural selection. This refers to how the animals which adapt best to the land before them grow strong and are more likely to reproduce. Therefore they will pass on their dominant characteristics to the next generation. As our forefathers lived in greatly differing environments e.g. the equator verses cold northern climates, humans have adapted to their environment and passed on these traits through many successive generations. The result is that any two people can differ in how their body reacts to any one particular way of "healthy living" (If you are a creationist then it is simply that God made us more unique than our current society would have us believe).

The evidence about how this influences human health started emerging in the 1920's when a dentist, Dr Weston A Price travelled the world to chart the nutrition, health and lifestyle of the different cultures around the world who were living off the land before them[8].

He found that there was a large variance in the types of natural diet eaten within the different cultures. He saw that the Eskimos ate a diet of almost exclusively protein and fats from seal, fish etc. Contrasting this were the tribal groups in South America who had an almost meat free diet. These two groups and many others in between these extremes had almost no cases of cancer, heart disease or mental illness. They had very little tooth decay despite not brushing their teeth and were what could be said to be 'in very good health'. Some suffered from minor illnesses but they were free from the degenerative diseases that afflict the West.

Dr Price also studied the effect on the health of these native cultures when they began to consume Western food. What he saw was that upon introduction to our food these native groups started to succumb to the same degenerative conditions prevalent in our society today. He went on to conclude that people had evolved to live off the foods before them through natural selection.

The different and individual nutritional needs we all have was further backed up by Dr Roger Williams in the 1950's through his book Biochemical individuality[1]. His work reviewed thousands of medical studies. He found that there was a large variety in almost every measure of the human body from organ size and shape to enzyme concentrations and effectiveness. Through his own studies and in review of many medical research studies he showed how vitamin and mineral requirements for individuals varied considerably. From this he coined the term, the Genotrophic approach to health. This states that if you fulfil your genetically inherited nutritional requirements you will optimize your health.

On a practical level you see biochemical individuality at work day in day out, we all have nose, ears, and eyes yet none of us look the same. It is for the same reason that your friends can eat whatever they want and not gain weight yet you cannot. This is because we are different on the inside and outside of the body. We all have the same enzymes, organs and structures but they vary greatly in size, shape and efficiency.

Biochemical individuality is everywhere in the world except in one place – It is not found in your health and fitness advice!!!! It is everywhere around you in every possible facet of the body except in the advice designed to make you healthy and look amazing! This is a major contributor to why the world is fat, unhealthy with no energy to do anything but watch TV. It is why there are five year old children who are overweight. If everyone truly understood how different and individual we are we would not have this culture of learned helplessness that dominates our society.

The reason most people do not do anything or try a different plan is that everyone is telling them that there is only one way to get results, e.g. follow the healthy eating guidelines etc. This advice is given by every institution from the government down to primary schools. So when someone fails to get results doing this methodology the immediate thought is not to adapt the plan, but rather to give up. The same applies to any expert that promotes a certain plan, e.g. low carb, high protein, long cardio. The reality is, it will probably work for some but not for others. You only need to worry about what works for you!

Taking an interest in getting results -

The reason that taking an interest is important is how it relates to knowledge and obtaining the knowledge that you need to get results. If you take no interest you will simply follow the crowd and do what they do. Now this would be great if the crowd had amazingly toned bodies and were energetic and healthy. Take a look out of the window and you will see a selection of overweight, unhappy, low energy people. The crowd is the last place you want to look for advice if you are serious about getting in shape.

Being interested in getting results is about searching for the answers to your problems. Taking an interest is not gossiping about what this celebrity did or what your best friend did. It is seeing how a piece of information affects you and getting results.

When taking an interest in getting results you need to become neutral and unemotional from the information.

Emotions are not too helpful when it comes to looking for the right answers. As humans we are amazing at seeing what we want to see. When your emotions are involved you will look for the information that supports your beliefs. When you are emotion free you are more likely to see the actual facts. It takes a high degree of true commitment to absorb information which may go against your beliefs. However, when it comes to health information this will be a frequent event.

If you want to get in shape then you can either carry on doing what you have always done, which, funnily enough will give you exactly the same if not worse results, or look to change your plan. However, if you take an interest in your results but do it through clouded glasses you will simply convince yourself you were right about everything. It will not change the facts for the body and the results (or lack of) will tell you the real story. Forget your existing beliefs, remove your emotions and start to discover and do the necessary actions to get results. This may go against what you have learnt previously, you may not like the answers and it may go against what the experts say. The question is do you want to be in amazing shape?

Many people will cite some reason why they are not interested in getting results. These excuses are just their way of rationalising a lack of success, either you know how to get results and you achieve it, or you do not. The remainder is just a story made up to amuse your mind but does not change the outcome.

You may say it is too hard to understand the information or every one contradicts each other, this is true. You may say, I do not understand nutrition, exercise isn't for me, I am not sure how it applies to me, I am too busy to find out how to lose weight, it is my doctors / trainers / friends responsibility to tell me what it takes to get results. The reality is you have all the abilities you need and you are the only one who can get results for yourself. While experts can guide you along the path they cannot carry you.

It does not require great intelligence when looking to find out and apply the information you need for results. The information for success can be understood by anyone. This is because success depends upon body awareness. This form of intelligence is far removed from the academic intelligence we traditionally think of. You will need to learn what to eat, what not to eat, how you feel after eating, what to do in an exercise session, how does it make you feel etc. It includes monitoring how your health changes. This has nothing to do with intelligence, you do not need to know statistics about foods and exercise, you simply need to know what, when and how to do it.

You should be taking an interest in food, what is in food, how it is prepared, how to cook, what your body needs, how it is different to other people, the various ways to exercise, injury prevention, injury rehabilitation, your mind, behaviour change, handling emotions, how other people handle the same problems you face and more. People in amazing shape know about these things. The list may seem intimidating but it does not take more than just a few minutes reading a day to develop this knowledge. It is no different to reading this book!

Finding the right information and people to help you –

When it comes to finding the right information you have to be very careful about the source of the information, the claims it makes and methodology it is based upon. You should also consider the implications of any plan on yourself regardless of how many other people have done well on it from the general population.

When it comes to information let's get one thing clear, there is a vast amount of information available, the problem is that everyone contradicts each other and you can find convincing arguments for many conflicting points of view. Most of societies' beliefs as a whole are simply a reflection of which view has been pushed the most. This is often as a result of a large publicity campaigns to promote them.

Take a look at the issue of smoking, just a few decades ago it was being promoted by doctors in TV adverts saying this is good for your health. Why were doctors promoting this? It was because they were paid some good money, but also because the cigarette companies had paid even better money to ensure research studies did not produce any adverse reports about the dangers of smoking. It took

30-40 years to turn around this viewpoint. Why do you think human psyche has changed since? Humans and society are the same. The only changes are the topics about which we are told false information. Where yesterday was smoking today it is your food.

When looking at society as a whole, is it full of people who are in great shape, good energy, great health with peace of mind? We are not even close and only getting further away. This is because the mainstream advice is wrong. Where does the advice you follow come from? If it stems down from the government then do not think this has to be the best quality information. The government advice is sponsored by big business.

While on your quest to get into shape you will need to be careful about which sources you use for information. For every good source there will be 5 to 10 sources of dreadful information. You need to be mindful of this.

You can of course use a health professional which is a great idea, but there are a few things to take into consideration. When choosing who to work with you should understand what aspect they cover and how it relates to your goals. Any long term results plan will need your mindset, nutrition and exercise plan to be in order. Many practitioners cover one small element of "health" which is great alongside other methods but redundant without other aspects being implemented. You should address your mind and nutrition first.

When working with a health professional or trainer you need to know what aspects you are covering with them. How are you covering the other aspects needed for results? Another important question to ask is - how does this relate in the long term picture? For example, you could make some great progress, say with counselling sessions but do you need to go for the rest of your life? Any long term plan must have you at a self sustainable level within a reasonable amount of time.

Whoever you work with and whatever role they play everything must be measured against the backdrop of results. Evaluate and react accordingly. If results are not forth coming do you need to bring in other techniques? Go deeper into biochemistry functioning? Or is the plan simply wrong? When viewing everything that you do against your results you will be able to monitor progress and react appropriately.

BEHAVIOUR CHANGE EXERCISES

Awareness –

Begin to start noticing the amazing difference between us all. Ask your friends about hunger, how they feel after eating certain foods and compare it to how you react. Take note of the many differences there are between you and your friends, e.g. who is more mathematical, musical, stronger, fitter etc

Start noticing the many contradictions in the media, notice the experts focusing on only one facet of health, yet claiming the grand solution. Just begin to observe the world around you and you will soon see what is clear for everyone to see, yet often goes unnoticed. We are all individuals, there is no one size fits all approach and most people are going about it all wrong. Sad but true! Try doing this for the next few days.

Questioning –

What beliefs do you have that are applied to the whole population and not the individual? How do you know the belief affects you the same way it does everyone else? What would it take for you to change your beliefs over to a tailored approach to getting results?

Intention

From today forward understand how special and different you are from everyone else around you. Touch your hand on your heart and say out loud ten times:

"I am totally unique! I am obsessed about finding out what my body needs to be in amazing shape"

Planning –

Try reading the material referenced in the appendix to learn more about individual approaches to nutrition, exercise and even the mind. Join my weekly newsletter at www.benwilsonuk.com

Emotional management –

How are your emotions affecting your view of the real information and facts out there? For example, are you following a low fat diet yet not losing weight and feeling hungry? If so, are you ignoring these facts because you have a fear of fat? It could be your emotional attachment to your favourite food is clouding your judgment about how it affects you badly. The body is tuned for success and knows what it needs. Forget the emotions and ask yourself what does my body really need?

PRINCIPLE 7 – ATTAIN BALANCE IN LIFE AND HAVE THE BEST OF BOTH WORLDS

People in amazing shape are very good at attaining a balance within all of their health and fitness behaviours. This allows them to follow their plan of action without resentment or feeling restricted. People who achieve long term success in their goals have also found a way to have the best of both worlds in what appears to be an either / or situation.

When it comes to creating balance in any health and fitness behaviour you will always struggle to achieve this if the behaviour is underpinned by emotions. For example, it is much more difficult to limit a food if you believe it makes you happy. If you are under too much stress and your primary coping mechanism is to eat or drink then it is hard to obtain a balance without addressing the underlying emotions and stress. However, when you have addressed the underlying emotions you will be able to achieve the level of balance that most people want to create with their eating and lifestyle.

Creating balance within your health and fitness behaviours comes in many forms. The main ways to create balance is outlined below. Different people in amazing shape will rely on some of the techniques below more than the others. The key is how you put it together to create that ideal level of balance. Remember that the most important factor to creating balance is by first removing the emotional foundations to the behaviour.

Strict periods, relaxed periods,

Most people in sensational shape go through a few periods a year where they are "strict" and get into even better shape than usual. This counters other periods where they are more "relaxed". As many people who are in amazing shape have a sporting background they are used to this cycle e.g. off season, pre season, in-season. It is just now the cycle has changed to pre holiday, pre Christmas, New Year etc.

Most out of shape people put in a poor effort in the New Year and an equally limp effort in their pre holiday phase. In fact, an out of shape person's best effort usually falls below the level of a relaxed period of someone in amazing shape.

People in great shape have relaxed periods but they always follow it with a period where they try to get into extraordinary shape. It is the time when the guy or girl in great shape clicks their fingers and says "I am into this" and starts making it happen. This is when they turn it up a notch. That is not to say while not going 100% they were doing everything wrong, but simply they were not doing everything right. It is natural to not go 100% all year round.

Balancing good meals versus bad ones

Almost all people in great shape balance their meals. It could be they know they are going out for a Pizza so that they ensure the meals earlier in the day are perfect and likewise the next day in compensation. They do this because they want to help their body out.

Conversely they do actually just eat the Pizza when they go out instead of trying to convince themselves that a pizza can be made healthy by having just two slices and a load of lettuce on the side. This is where out of shape people let themselves down. They do not balance the meals before and after and then they try to be 'good' when they are out in a restaurant. The result is they feel deprived and restricted all the time.

Other examples are where people worry at the beach about whether to eat an ice cream. It is not worth worrying about it if you go to the beach a few times a year. One meal here or there is absolutely irrelevant. Contrast that with putting that focus into really working on breakfasts and lunches every other day of the year. If you live in Spain on the beach however, this behaviour would need to be examined if it continued to happen day in day out.

The breakfast effect

This refers to the importance of a regular meal such as breakfast compared to what you do on a Saturday night. People who are out of shape will almost always focus on how they had one meal out in a restaurant or that they had one or two bits of chocolate during the week. They focus on this while ignoring what they ate for breakfast and lunch each day. This shows an imbalance in their approach. If you eat 21 meals a week how can you blame that one dinner out on not getting results? This is exactly what the overweight person does. He/she blames that one meal instead of taking the time to address their regular 9am - 5pm meals.

To me breakfast is the most important meal of the day. It sets the tempo for the day ahead. Breakfasts are almost always free from social influences and have much less emotional ties. They also comprise up to a third of your weeks meals. You cannot afford to get this wrong.

Western society has a bowl of cereal for breakfast and a more typical 'meal' for dinner. Did you ever ask yourself why this is the case? Why do we not have it the other way round? Why do we not have cereal for dinner instead of breakfast? I have been to China, Malaysia and many other countries where this is not the case. I have seen rice dishes, curry, raw fish and many other foods eaten for breakfast. If we lived in a cave would we have different foods for breakfast than dinner? The reason we are cereal based at breakfast time is all to do with advertising and little to do with nutritional facts.

My breakfasts are identical to evening meals. If you eat meat and vegetables for dinner then why not for breakfast? When I discuss this topic I almost invariably find that out of shape people look on in horror of choosing any other food but their bowl of cereal. However, how can you afford to get seven meals a week totally wrong and then demand you get results and be in awesome shape? For many people this is exactly what they are doing. Breakfast should be one of the very first places you visit on your quest for results because for a large percentage of people cereal will not allow for results.

If you want balance in your life and not need to worry about your eating when out in a restaurant then it can often be achieved simply by ensuring your breakfasts and lunches are perfect. This will guarantee at least two thirds of your weekly meals are in place.

Bad behaviours tempered by good behaviours

People in amazing shape are pretty good at creating some level of balance between their behaviours. When they know they are going to splurge in the evening they back it up with 100% good eating during the day and the next morning afterwards. They are making a trade off. People in poor shape look to have their cake and eat it.

If the person in great shape knows they cannot train next week because of a work trip they train the two days before they leave and two days after they get back. They are trading fitness to great effect. The average person in awful shape dreads the thought of doing any exercise and uses the trip as another great reason why they tried their best but couldn't exercise again this month. Alternatively it could be that someone in shape has been out drinking a few nights one week. They counter this by having a week without alcohol. When it comes to tempering bad behaviours with good ones the biggest key is that you trade like for like behaviours.

Trading like for like behaviours

One of the most important things to be aware of is how you trade behaviours. You can only trade behaviours that are of the same type. If you eat badly for a period it must be traded with a period of good eating. If you miss your exercise routine then it must be traded with some exercise sessions later on. You cannot trade different behaviours! This is where most gym goers go dramatically wrong. They believe by exercising it will account for their poor eating. This is not how the body works. If you were trying to train for a marathon do you think you could just eat good meals without going for a run? The same applies in reverse and especially for weight loss. You cannot trade different behaviours.

People do this trying to trade calories for exercise. However, the numbers are heavily stacked against you in terms of food vs exercise. You can eat an hour's worth of exercise in minutes. It is a dangerous game to play and thus you should only trade bad eating for a period of good eating.

This is not to say you shouldn't exercise if you are eating badly but if you spend a week eating rubbish you will probably need to put in a week of eating really well. If you pig out in a restaurant then that's fine but do not think a gym session is an equal trade, it is not! You must eat maybe two perfect meals to trade it off.

I run an athletics group. It is amazing to see how many people come down and do an awesome session of tough sprints and then say something like 'great, now I can eat some junk food this weekend' This is a poor attitude to have. They could have saved the effort of the track by just eating right all weekend and not training. Obviously they would miss out on the fitness benefits but if the main goal is fat loss the nutrition element will always be the most important.

Balance in exercise

Exercise can be summed up by the word consistency. This is the one crucial element to produce results. If you start, then stop, then start again you will never find you progress much. People in great shape achieve consistency in exercise because for one thing they have learnt how to enjoy it (notice I said learnt, anyone, including you, can learn to enjoy it) and they know how to achieve balance in their routine

The way to exercise consistently is to allow yourself to have both intense periods of training followed by easier training periods. This is exactly what professional athletes do. They do not train equally as hard during the whole training year. Instead they have a rest period (off-season), a high intensity period (pre season) and then a moderate period so their body is fresh for competition (playing season). All exercisers should use a rotation of some kind.

The out of shape person either falls into having a year round off season or they go intensely for too long and then fall off. I would urge you to train for a sport. This gives you a level of focus that you cannot replicate elsewhere and takes away any resentment in having to do exercise. It also allows you to plan periods of exercise intensity and relief. A point to note is that during a relief period you still do some exercise but at lower levels and in lesser amounts.

The same concept applies to training sessions. Some workouts are easy others are hard. Most people turn up every session expecting personal bests. This is ridiculous if you understand how the body works. Look to tune into how you feel before an exercise session and decide to go easier some days compared to others.

If you usually run twenty minutes at speed 11 on the treadmill but you come in the gym feeling a bit drained you instead run 10 minutes at speed 9.5. This easier session will re-energise you. What most people do is instead get put off by the thought of going hard at speed 11 and make up an excuse not to go. If you lifted 20Kg for 10 reps Monday then maybe Wednesday you lift 12.5 Kg for the 10 reps instead.

In your mind you must understand there is no minimum time or intensity for an exercise session. When you truly believe this you will never struggle with exercise again. This is because you will have knocked out the two biggest excuses why you do not do it, e.g. I haven't enough time or cannot be bothered with the effort. If you are someone who does not exercise then you will need to examine the blocks to why you have not started a programme. Once you are comfortable exercising then observing the no minimum time or effort rule will keep you on track.

Binge eating

Many people have a problem with binge eating. Typically there are two main causes. One of these is just an overload of emotions that you try to mask with food. These excessive emotions usually coincide with a loss of hope. The second reason is a perception that you have blown it now so you may as well do whatever you want. These two reasons normally always come hand in hand with each other and are exacerbated if you are simultaneously experiencing some of the different types of hunger. As ever, emotional anchors to the foods eaten in a binge will further heap more negative behaviours into the situation.

If you have attained true balance within your behaviours the "I have blown it now" reasons for binge eating disappear. You do not feel restricted so there is no need to blow off steam when your 'self enforced restriction' is broken.

Binge eating is worsened by the belief "I will never eat this food again (after this binge)". This creates a panic internally so you eat as much of that food as possible before "quitting" for life. It is more productive to tell yourself "I will have it again sometime in the future and it is ok to do this. I have had enough for now". This is the concept of true balance in relation to your foods. You are free enough to eat any food yet strict enough to naturally not want to consume it above the threshold that prevents results.

If you do have an episode of binge eating then it is important to not beat yourself up or make negative statements about who you are as a person. Simply observe and try to get to the bottom of the problem. I would start with trying to reduce your overall level of emotions. Persistent binge eating can also be caused by simply consuming too few calories for what your body needs and/or too little carbohydrates.

Meal by meal and food by food analysis

If you review your progress of eating by a daily or weekly time period you leave yourself open to becoming demoralised. If you judge yourself on a daily basis and then have a terrible breakfast you immediately think that today is already a failure. This will greatly decrease your motivation for the rest of the day and could even be enough to start off an episode of binge eating if other factors are also present.

Weekly reviewing also leaves you open to periods of poor eating. When you know you can't get a good week after messing up a day then you may decide to start again the week afterwards and eat poorly in the meantime. Even a good weeks eating can cause problems because you may decide to 'reward' yourself and go crazy on the weekend. This is especially troublesome if you are not trading like behaviours as discussed earlier.

The most effective method for evaluating your eating is on a meal by meal or even food by food basis. I have discussed how one meal cannot do any harm in the long run which is true, but at the same time any week is made up of 20 plus individual meals. Therefore you will find success easier if you take a meal by meal judgement only.

Almost everyone who is trying to get into shape has some sort of measurement timescale they use whether it is consciously or subconsciously. It is important to have this but if you switch to a meal on meal basis only from your current evaluation, then it raises the bar. When you judge progress at each meal there is no room for writing off a day or a week because you messed up, there is also no time to go crazy because you have been so good recently.

Judge each meal on its own merits then move on. If you have a great meal, then celebrate its success. Feel happy you just got a meal spot on. Be proud of your efforts. Do this each time you eat a good meal. The more you celebrate, the greater the desire to get each meal right becomes. All of sudden you want to get a meal right because of the good feeling you will receive.

Some people like to reward themselves for getting a good meal right. This should never ever be in the form of some other food. As what does this tell you? It says that this food is somehow superior, what you truly wanted. Attaining balance in your life is never about rewarding yourself with some rubbish food because you ate well for a meal or two.

If you have run a few good meals together you may begin to judge yourself on the daily or weekly progress. Avoid doing this, judge each meal individually and forget about the daily or weekly progress. It just sets you up for things to go wrong.

But how do I attain balance if I do not judge a weekly overview you may ask? Well this is just the point, when you are not connected to the food you will not need to actively seek out balancing the behaviour, instead it happens naturally. Judge yourself meal by meal and then look at your results. That will tell you everything else you need to know about balance.

Having both options in your life

Another way people who are in amazing shape act differently from their overweight counterparts is how they see that they can almost invariably have both options within an either / or situation. They can both go out for dinner and be in shape, they can be both find time for exercise and their family, they can have the social life they want and still only drink moderately. The ability to have both options is one of the most powerful ways to negate the reasons most out of shape people will cite for not doing a certain behaviour.

Invariably there is almost no situation which cannot be created alongside being in shape. If you are thinking, "but I want to eat as much chocolate as I can and be in shape" then even that can be achieved. You can keep the "eat as much chocolate as you want" attitude but just change your desire so you naturally only want a small amount. Then you have got both. The way to do this is by getting as much pleasure and happiness from other sources so that your desire to eat the chocolate is naturally reduced. The world of having both options is easily attainable if you have removed the emotional connections to the behaviours in question.

It is easy to only have junk food once or twice a week if it is not your emotional support, it is easy to say no in a dinner party if you do not have an emotional craving for the food, you can avoid getting drunk at a work event if you not feeling pressurised (note it is you who creates the pressure feeling and not other people). Exercise is easy to find time for if you feel only enjoyment and excitement from it. You can have just a slice or two of cake if you do not feel uncomfortable at the party and you could easily pass on the biscuits when you know it does not make you happy. The only way to achieve this balance is to get to the stage of not needing it emotionally.

Long term, if you try to give up something to get in shape it may become a struggle. Instead you should look for ways to have balance within your behaviours while looking at ways to attain the best of both worlds. It is certainly possible to stop a behaviour in the short term but if you fail to do the emotional work around it then it will rarely work in the longer term. I know clients who gave up going out for a few months so they could lose weight. How could this ever work? They were pitting their social life versus being in shape. The strategy was doomed to failure and was unnecessary for results. The solution is always to find a way to do both, to keep the social part yet still do it with the balance that allows you to get all the benefits without the negatives. Try suggesting to friends to go bowling instead of boozing, to meet at the tennis club or park instead of the coffee shop or café. The options are endless. The biggest obstacle is always your own emotionally based views which cloud you from seeing the solution.

BEHAVIOUR CHANGE EXERCISES

Awareness –

Consider which areas of your health and fitness do you obtain a good balance and which are out of balance? Spend time contemplating what degree of balance you have within your – breakfasts, lunches, dinners, eating out, drinking water, eating chocolate/sweets, eating other junk food, exercise, drinking alcohol. Include others that may apply to you.

Questioning –

Why are some of your behaviours in balance? Why are other behaviours out of balance? What would it take for you to create balance in all your behaviours?

Intention

Decide to create balance within the different areas of your life. Touch your hand on your heart and say out loud Ten times:

"I maintain a perfect balance between the behaviours needed to achieve my results and living the life I want to lead"

Planning –

Look at the areas where you have an imbalance within your behaviours. Plan out how you could trade off and create balance in this area. Remember you cannot trade different behaviours, e.g. a heavy night of drinking cannot be traded for an exercise session. Heavy drinking can only be traded for a period of lesser drinking at some point.

If you find all your behaviours are in balance yet you are not getting results then you are either following the wrong plan, have not resolved blocking factors or your emotions have set the level of balanced behaviours above the threshold for results.

Emotional management –

For the areas that are out of balance it is more than likely you have an underlying emotional belief fuelling this behaviour. Can you identify it?

From now on whenever you do the activity that is out of balance I want you to say to yourself "This gives me nothing emotionally". Say it to yourself each time you take a drink, eat that chocolate or cake. You do not have to change the behaviour but you do need to tell yourself it gives you nothing emotionally. Over time it will begin to knock away at your belief system. While doing the out of balance activity ask yourself how else can you fulfil the underlying emotional need? Look for evidence to support you.

PRINCIPLE 8 – ASSOCIATE WITH OTHERS IN AMAZING SHAPE

One of the most effective ways to get yourself heading in the right direction is through becoming friends with people who are already where you want to get to. Who you associate with has a huge influence upon the likely success of your progress. It is not that you need to disown all your current friends but it is a case of maybe finding one or two new ones who are exactly where you want to be.

You will recall that one of the biggest ways we learn our behaviours is by simply copying what we see. One of the most effective ways for you to make progress after finishing this book is to find one or more friends who are in amazing shape. This could come in the form of joining an exercise group, hiring a personal trainer or spending more time with your friend who is the 'healthy one' in your social group.

When it comes to who you associate with it is pretty much impossible to only spend time with people in amazing shape, nor is it that necessary. It would be an unhealthy way to live life. Someone who is in good shape is not better or worse than those who are out of shape, they simply have better subconscious programmes when it comes to food and health. The key is to not let people drag you down within your health and fitness behaviour. To do this you should become aware of the different fitness personalities.

Once you are aware of someone's fitness personality you are able to filter the information and influences they have upon you. There are five fitness personality types. You have already encountered one which is fake thin people. If you know someone is a fake thin person you should treat their advice very differently to someone who is in amazing shape. It is not that you should stop being friends, but simply view their advice differently. The other four main fitness personality types are:

Out of shape people who do not care about it

This group of people are the ones who have no apparent interest in their health and are living in blissful ignorance. Well, this is blissful if you consider having no energy, poor health, mental unease and various health symptoms a blissful experience. Their views are littered with blocking beliefs, unhelpful behaviour patterns and will simply reflect general society or follow the trend from what they have recently read or seen on TV.

People who are not interested in their health will be the ones who do nothing in regards to diet and exercise. These people will have a negative influence on you in general but at the same time you must be very used to them because they are ten a dozen. This is your average person.

If this person is in your family then they can be unsupportive in that they will question why are you always doing this diet or that and why are you exercising etc. The key thing for you to know they have a very different viewpoint on health related issues.

People who have no interest in health will only repeat common knowledge and loosely held beliefs. Simply treat these comments with passing attention and let them go on by.

Many of these people can be very helpful and supportive. For these people the same rules apply. Focus on yourself, get that in order and lead by being the change. This is an important point, we often find it is easier to try and change someone else in the hope that it would then make it easier for us or because they need it so much more. This is probably very true but every other person is irrelevant to your health. I had a client once who said "you had better not be going away eating pizzas while I am doing this". This is a totally unrelated piece of information. If I am eating 10 pizzas a day you are still the same size, if I do not eat any pizza you are still the same size! End of story.

So instead of trying to help others who are in this stage I would simply focus on achieving your own goals and in time they may be inspired by your success to change themselves.

Out of shape people who are trying to be in shape but failing

This type of person has the potential to be the very worst to associate with. The people who do not care about health do not warrant any of your attention on health issues. The people who are trying to get in shape are in a similar category as you and thus you will look to them for support and advice etc. Sadly, if they are failing then their advice is no more helpful than the ones who have not even tried. Whilst effort is commendable it is about actions and results!

This type of person can make life difficult for you because they will usually burden you with how hard everything is, how much they want to eat some chocolate, how hard it is to motivate themselves, how they hate exercise, how their body hurts, their medical conditions. They will recite almost all of the blocking beliefs I have outlined previously.

This can be disastrous because as you begin your journey you will be starting to see, feel and truly understand the points I have outlined here and you will begin behaving exactly like a person in amazing shape. As things progress you can then bump into your failing friend who then burdens you with their problems and before you know it you have slipped back into your old ways. It is common to slip back into old ways. The key is how quickly you snap straight back out of it! When around other failing people they can prolong the time it takes to snap back out of it or even prevent it from happening.

As you now know, when achieving balance in your life it is not about avoiding these people per se. It is about ensuring you have a selection of the different fitness personalities and reframing your mind set in how you deal with them. At the end of the day they are trying their best to achieve their goals but through a lack of knowledge and application they are not achieving them. What you need to do is start to look out for the mistakes they are making. This will meant any time spent with them is increasing your awareness.

A point to note is the mistakes they keep making are probably the very same ones you are (were) doing. In fact, you have probably copied each other. So do not judge people for their mistakes as they are doing their best with what they know and have been through so far, so simply observe and learn.

Out of shape people who are succeeding and getting into shape

The previous categories are not the people you should copy in behaviour but rather they are to be used to help increase your own awareness of your faulty behaviour patterns.

This fitness personality type is where you want to be. Depending where and when they started their journey they may be looking great already or simply much better than a few weeks / months back. Either way, they are doing something right and you want to see how they have done it. This does not mean you will copy them because it is working for their body, instead you will gather information about how they have done it and use what applies to you and then discard what does not.

The people in this stage are very enthusiastic and are great to hang out with. They are on form and wanting to keep things going. If possible you should look to spend time with them and try to do mutual activities together. For example, going to the supermarket with someone in great shape or is getting into great shape can often help you avoid the awful foods that litter the aisles.

In this category you must be aware of the person you are listening to again. Remember different people can lose weight / get in shape in different ways. Their method may not be an efficient way for you to lose weight. At the same time watch out for Yo-Yo dieters. They will go through all three stages in a fairly predictable pattern of behaviour. They will have a period of not caring, then they will try something and fail, then they will get switched on (often due to a holiday, wedding or similar external goal) and achieve fat loss during that time before allowing themselves to regain the lost weight back. You should classify these people as out of shape failing because their methods do not work long term. However, they may appear as this fitness personality type when you meet them.

People in amazing shape –

The final group are the ones to respect in regards to their health and fitness. These are the ones who are exactly where you want to be. They have put in place a system and behaviour pattern to produce some remarkable results. Assuming they are not fake thin people, then every minute spent with them will be helping you.

It should be noted there are a lot of fake thin people who look great. Treat them as you would the other categories. Observe and listen to their mistakes and then ask yourself are you making these too? Simultaneously, look out for things that may work for you and incorporate these into your behaviours.

This is why it is important to never take anyone's word as gospel. You need to extract the information that can be beneficial to you and then discard that which is not applicable. This is true even from people truly in amazing shape. Some of things they do may not work for you.

Show no resentment to people already in amazing shape

It is quite common to see various forms of resentment towards people in sensational shape and you will often assume many generalisations which are not true. The long and the short of it is this: "You can never become something that you resent". How could you? Your subconscious would never allow it. If you think people in amazing shape are arrogant and you do not like arrogant people, you will never go onto to achieve your goal for fear of being seen as arrogant. If you think people in amazing shape are rude, strict, unfriendly, intimidating, show off's etc then these are all negative beliefs about the very goal to which you are trying to aspire. They could be big enough beliefs to stop the subconscious allowing you to get there. This may seem illogical, but the human mind can often act that way.

You must incorporate and replace any negative views you have of people in amazing shape with positive ones. The major reason for most negative views is from nasty experiences with fake thin people and false assumptions you have made as a result.

When you move beyond resenting people who are already where you want to be you will find yourself really keen to meet these types of people and learn from them. If you resent people like this you will try to avoid them.

Achieving a balance in your associates

As you can see from the above there is absolutely no one you need to fear or to avoid spending time with. In fact, I would encourage you to have a selection of friends from all four categories. What you must do though is be sure that you know roughly what type of person everyone is and then just be an observer. With everything you see direct it inwards and consider your own behaviours and then use these answers to improve your results.

Using this approach you will find even the most pushy of friends encouraging you to eat some cake will barely have an effect. It will instead give you some great feedback. You will ask why is he/she pushing this cake onto me? Why do I feel tempted? Any feedback is great feedback!

If you do not have any friends or family members in any one of the four categories then you should really get on the lookout for this sort of person. In general I find it hard to believe you will not know anyone who doesn't care about their health or struggles to achieve the results they desire. They are everywhere. The other two types may not be in your social circle yet. You can find these people everywhere but you just need to look for them. Exercise groups are always a good place to start.

Initially when you do not have many acquaintances who are in amazing shape you should be on the lookout for a subtle lowering of your own standards. When you see how "normal" people act you may think that because you are doing so much more than them you are doing well. This is true in part but your behaviours may still fall way below the levels of people who are in truly amazing shape.

Confusing successful people in life for successful people in health and fitness

One thing I have noticed over the years is how people who are very successful in one area are given undue credit for their knowledge in another. Just because you have built a very successful business it does not count for anything in terms of health and fitness. Just because someone has a PhD, is well read on current affairs, is amazing at pub quizzes or is on TV, it does not mean they have any special authority on health and fitness.

Often, successful people in business or their careers are very head strong and opinionated. This can easily lead you to conclude that because they know a lot about their field they must also know more than you on the issue of health and fitness. This is not true! The only way someone should be judged is on their health and fitness is through the degree of success they have achieved.

Partnering or teaming up

A common approach to losing weight is teaming up with a partner and / or going to a club or group. This approach has potentially both good and bad points to it. Making a commitment to someone else is very powerful. In general most people will put in more effort in order to not let someone else down than they would to not let themselves down.

This is where a training partner or group of people can be very helpful. It is also good if you are competitive. The desire to beat someone is a very powerful human emotion. It can drive men and women to amazing levels of commitment, focus and success.

The downside of this is that being committed to someone who can potentially drag you down can make life much more difficult. When you make a commitment to someone else and vice versa you also may have the problem of what to do when someone breaks the pact. If you are the one who breaks it then you may really beat yourself up which might just lead to you eating plenty of poor quality foods for comfort (a pointless strategy as you must know by now). Alternatively, if they break the pact then you may think it gives you permission to go off the rails as well.

When it comes to competition, it certainly drives things forward, but relying on an external stimulus of which you have no control can lead you in the wrong direction. Another problem with competition is no one likes losing and if you can see you cannot win, then sometimes this puts you off from trying.

In short, partnering and teaming up is more efficient than doing it alone IF, and only IF, you set it up in the right way. If you are teaming up with someone you must know exactly where they are classified in terms of their fitness personality. They should inspire you to a higher level and not pull you down. Even then, the arrangement should be two individuals working on their goals but in close alignment. This means that with or without them you are doing your plan. If they start to reduce your motivation and inspiration then look to dissolve the alliance.

Dealing with specific people

Often you may find that there is just one person that seems to prevent you attaining success and / or acting how you want. This invariably is your partner, best friend or close family member etc. This is an issue you must address. There are two things that you must do, first ask yourself, why are they acting this way? Then classify them along the lines of their health and fitness personality type. Bear in mind every-body acts a certain way for a reason. It is rarely to be nasty to you but bears out of their beliefs, fears and best wishes for you and them.

When you are dealing with one of the closest people to you then you may find some contradictions from other similar health and fitness personalities you will meet. For example, have you noticed just how much less patience you have with your parents on almost any issue compared to other people? This is because of the past you have shared together. When they say something reasonable you may interpret it as the 1000th bit of nagging you have heard over the last ten years. When a new person says exactly the same thing you have all the time in the world to hear their story.

The result of this is that your partner may appear to nag at you instead of supporting you in a way he/she would support their best friend. This could simply be because of the way you interpret their advice. Alternatively, they may not treat you the same because they want you to succeed so much more than with their friends. Perhaps he/she is so much more worried about your health than their friends they end up hindering your efforts rather than helping. Emotions make people act differently and often inefficiently. Your partner and parents etc may say something which you perceive as nasty but it is just because they care so much and that is the only way that they know how to "motivate you".

Once you have identified the influence of your closest relationships in regards to your goals you must then create a solution to go forwards. This will of course depend upon the influences on you.

In my experience the influence of your partner or parents is not normally a huge problem if it is not against the back drop of your own emotional connections to the negative behaviours. If your partner buys you a chocolate bar because he/she thinks it makes you happy and you agree with this belief then you may cite this present as an excuse to eat it. If you didn't hold these beliefs about chocolate your partner would not have bought it, or if they did you would not have been tempted by it.

If your behaviour changes cause friction or you find the person is highly persistent in trying to knock you off track then it means they are feeling threatened or worried that they are missing out on something because of your changes. It could also be because they now feel pressured as well to do this action.

To overcome this you will need to ease their concerns. You can do this by reassuring them you will not change in a negative way. Tell them you will still be the same person. Let them know they can keep their habits and do not need to do the same changes.

I can understand this fear shown by partners, friends and family alike. If one of their favourite pleasures is going out for meals with you they will feel threatened when you tell them that you no longer eat rubbish food. If they use chocolate to try to de-stress they may feel exposed as you declare that it does not help you at all emotionally. Your partner may even go so far as to fear that as you look better you may leave them.

It is possible that your behaviour may make them feel bad about how they act. After declaring you do not drink your friends may all be worried that they will look stupid because you are watching them while sober. These are just a few of the many fears that your closest acquaintances may think. Do try and bear in mind that they are human. They are as illogical and emotional as you and I are. They are just acting naturally and doing their best.

The solution to this is never too difficult. The golden rule is always to change yourself only and not the other person. Then you need to protect and maintain what they stand to lose. You can usually find a way to attain a balance and find a compromise that allows them to still get what they wanted and for you to get the results you want.

If the issue is going out for dinner, then agree on a certain frequency or go to restaurants where you can eat a good meal (remember the Breakfast effect). If it is about giving up a food then do not nag them to not eat it but instead repeat the fact that it may be fine for them but not for you. If it is alcohol then still go to exactly the same places but stay sober and just do your own thing. Do not remind everyone the next time you see them saying how drunk they were, let them do that to each other. Whatever their fears, simply alleviate them, in doing so strike a balance so that you both can get what you want.

If part of your inspiration to change is to get the people closest to you to change, then you must do this by inspiring them through your behaviours and not by nagging, commenting, sniping and generally having a go at them. If they ask for help, then great, but even then give advice cautiously and just discuss how you act. When it comes to changing the people closest to you there is a fair chance they will not listen to you even if you are the top expert in the country. This is because they know you, your past and generally have a tougher time accepting what you say. The only way to really get them to listen is by showing them the proof.

In general you are better off directing them to someone else, be it a friend or expert who says the same thing you are trying to tell them. They are many times more likely to change behaviour from listening to them rather than you. If possible you can always swap with your friends so you help each others' partners etc.

BEHAVIOUR CHANGE EXERCISES

Awareness –

Classify your friends and acquaintances within the five main fitness personality types:

- Out of shape and do not care.
- Out of shape and failing.
- Out of shape and succeeding,
- Fake thin people
- People in amazing shape.

Questioning –

What personality type are most of the people you spend your time with? How do you let them influence you? How can you find more people in amazing shape to spend time with?

Intention

Decide from today that you now use all your friends as inspiration, whether they are winning or losing the game of health and fitness. Touch your hand on your heart and say out loud ten times:

"I actively seek out friends who are in amazing shape, I learn from my friends whatever shape they are in"

Planning –

Take a few moments to plan how you will deal with the various people in your life. Remember that other people's influence is much greater when it is anchoring into your own beliefs, e.g. the chocolate is only tempting if you think it is giving you something. Plan out how you will treat your closest acquaintances.

Actively seek out people in amazing shape. Check out my website for links to groups, trainers and communities (www.benwilsonuk.com). Make a plan to find some new friends in amazing shape.

Emotional management –

Look to use your friends to charge you emotionally. I find I am as charged up by people in awful shape as much as those in great shape. When you see someone eating junk food tune into how this makes you feel. If you are feeling a longing for their food say to yourself "Food gives me nothing emotionally". If your friends give you good ideas then copy these and incorporate them into your life.

When you are with someone in great shape then just feed off them. Remind yourself this is where you deserve to be. At the same time, look out for any resentment feelings. This can impede you getting results. Always be aware of the balance factor. If you meet someone in awesome shape eating a big dinner and having some drinks you may immediately think "that is so unfair, he/she can eat what she likes and still look great" However, you do not know if he/she has been perfect with every other meal for the last week and thus is perfectly entitled to do that or whether they are a fake thin person.

PRINCIPLE 9 – INCORPORATE THE AMAZING SHAPE ATTITUDES INTO YOUR PERSONALITY

I noticed a trend with my clients who got great results and those that didn't. The ones who got great results were fairly outgoing with telling the world about their new behaviours and acting differently in front of people. The people who got bad results would appear much more timid. They hoped by acting a certain way for a few weeks nobody would spot their changes before going back to being the same old person as before but having transformed their body.

Let's get this straight from the start, your current behaviours got you to where you are today. If you want long term results going forwards you are going to have change some behaviours and then maintain them long term.

There is no way in the world you can change something for just two months then return to your old patterns and expect the results to last. Why would that work? It doesn't! If your behaviour patterns worked in the first place you would not be in the position to need to change them to get results! This is crucial to understand, to get long term results you are going to have to change and keep these changes. For this to happen your behaviours must become part of your personality.

Many people do not want to tell the world about their new behaviours because they are worried they will be questioned on them, maybe they are afraid they will be seen as trying and failing yet again. Perhaps they do not want to put people out, look stupid, draw attention to themselves or one of the many other possible reasons. At some point though you have to let the world know about your new behaviours. Once the world understands these it will support you in doing them.

Another important reason for incorporating behaviours into your personality is because it sends a message to your brain. If you send mixed messages to your brain you will get mixed behaviour patterns back. Send clear messages to your brain and you get clear behaviour patterns back.

Every time you say you act a certain way it sends a direct signal to your subconscious. This cements and clarifies the behaviour patterns within you so that over time it goes from being a concentrated choice, to a natural choice to the only choice. When the new behaviour is the only choice to you that makes any sense, it will stay with you for life. This is what people in amazing shape have. The right behaviour patterns are naturally ingrained within them. Acting one way but telling the world you act another way doesn't influence the subconscious to create behaviour change.

People in amazing shape are known to other people by the behaviours they do. This is because they openly let people know that they act this way and they make no apologies for believing and doing what they do.

The goal for you is to become known for your health and fitness behaviours. When this happens you will be set for long term success. This is because your behaviour patterns will be set within your subconscious and thus you will be on automatic. It is not about only being known for your health and fitness behaviours but it is about other people treating you according to your values.

You wouldn't harass a Muslim in Ramadan to eat or drink during the day because you understand their religious views. The same view point should be taken from your friends. They shouldn't harass you about your behaviours if they understand what they are and how they are important to you.

When your personality is one that has good health and fitness behaviours running through it you will soon get some amazing results. It is at this point that other people will be very interested in what and why you do things. People in amazing shape have no problem telling others what they did to get there.

Incorporating the personality traits into you

One of the biggest difficulties in making behaviour changes is maintaining a level of emotional congruence when changing from a previous behaviour towards another path. For example, if you always criticised people following a diet and now you find yourself following a new nutrition routine (what some would call a diet) it can prove a block to wanting to put that change in place. It also causes you to not reveal your new behaviour to the world. This can be easily avoided by citing some good solid reasons for the new behaviours. When other people see your new behaviours are in keeping with your new beliefs (congruence) then there is never usually trouble in crossing over.

One way to do this is to cite results, you can usually dissolve all trouble by saying that since you have changed to _____ your body has improved in _____ way, e.g. since stopping bread I have lost two stone, since stopping alcohol I have felt much happier.

The biggest frictions I have seen in people's reactions when adopting new behaviours is when you still believe something yet you are changing your behaviours to one opposite to that belief. For example, if you believe 'I love eating rubbish food' yet you are on a diet, this is not a congruent belief. If you are tired of eating rubbish foods because it hurts your stomach so now you steer clear of the worst foods to upset your digestive system, you are showing some congruence. If you love going to the gym, no one will ever question you, if you hate it but go occasionally people will ask why you have a gym membership?

Any area in which you are being challenged will probably be an area you are not showing congruence within your beliefs. When you do show it people will just show inquisition.

Depending on your personality and social situation you may choose to make your changes in subtle and quiet way or in a very outgoing and loud way. There are no rights or wrongs as long as you show congruence and you do let the world know about your behaviour changes when pushed on them. You could announce to the world that you are to stop bread to see how it affects your body or simply stop without telling anyone and when offered a sandwich reveal why you are saying no.

As discussed previously it is always vital that you protect the interests of the other person when making your changes. This is to avoid friction and being pressured by them to cave in and return to your previous ways. To do this simply point out that they can still do the behaviour you have stopped e.g. I am no longer eating bread which means more to you!! As opposed to, none of us are eating bread because I am on a diet!

BEHAVIOUR CHANGE EXERCISES

Awareness –

What behaviours are you known for amongst your social group? Which ones of these would you like to keep and which would need to change for long term success?

Ask some of your closer friends how they would describe you in terms of health and fitness behaviours. If the answer is anything less than really health conscious or a health and fitness freak you will need to change some areas of your behaviours if you want long term success to be easy.

Questioning –

Why are you known for your current behaviours? Why are you not known for more productive behaviours? What would it take for you to change your beliefs over?

Intention

From today, begin incorporating the traits that will help you get results into your personality.

Start letting people in the world know what you are doing. Touch your hand on your heart and say out loud ten times:

"I am proud of my new behaviours and beliefs, I show them to the world and make no apologies for it"

Planning –

Focus on the areas that you will need to change for long term success. Identify if you are the kind of person who prefers to do things subtly or more significantly. Put in place a plan which acts in accordance with your personality style. For example, if you are a big drinker you could just declare you are stopping drinking, or maybe say you are cutting it out for a month, or more subtly just reduce your alcohol from 5 pints to 2 pints a night for a few weeks. Then reduce further, and so forth.

Remember how you can always have both when changing your behaviour. Think about how your new behaviour can be arranged to still give you both the benefits for your body and also serve the other purposes of that behaviour, e.g. be sociable, spend time with partner etc.

Put in place a plan of telling the world about all of your new behaviours. The more the world knows the new you the more likely change is to happen. Ensure you have emotional congruence as outlined below.

Emotional management –

For the areas that you are planning to change your behaviours look at your level of congruence. Spend time thinking about your beliefs up to this point, which includes how others may view your beliefs and then contrast this to the new behaviour patterns you want to create.

Think up a story that shows congruence between your new behaviours and beliefs so that you are not challenged by your friends and family as well as creating acceptance within your own mind. Allow for protecting the interests of other people in any planned changes.

For example, I saw on TV that in some people dairy can make them overweight and have skin issues. I decided to do an experiment and I have lost weight and my skin has improved. I must be one of those unlucky people who cannot eat it. All the more for you everyone else!

I always have hated exercise but I tried a sample personal training session. I absolutely loved it! It is so different to what I have done before. I think I might continue doing this and see if I can actually get into exercise.

PRINCIPE 10 – FOLLOW THE RIGHT PLAN FOR SUCCESS

When push comes to shove the margin of your success comes down to the quality of the plan you have and how closely you stick to it. However good your mind set may be you cannot ever get results if the plan of action you are sticking to is wrong. It is as simple as that.

Getting in amazing shape is a journey from point A to point B. If you have the right mind set you will be moving much faster, however, this is only beneficial if you are moving in the right direction i.e. you are following the right plan.

Every person in amazing shape has a plan of action that covers nutrition, exercise and motivation in some way, even if they are not aware of it themselves. The key thing is the plan works for them. If they didn't have this in place then they wouldn't have achieved the body they have. It is also important to note that just because one person is in shape using one system it has no bearing on whether this will work for you. This is because we are all unique in how our bodies work.

General advice fails more than it helps

The reason this is such an important element and one of the ten attitudes people in amazing shape have is because the general plan and advice for healthy living and getting into shape does not work for everyone. In truth it is worse than that, it does not work for the majority of people.

If it did work then everyone with just a little bit of motivation could follow it come the New Year and be in amazing shape by the summer. This does not happen because the general advice is wrong and almost every plan is never accompanied by looking at the faulty mind set.

If the general advice of losing weight worked then the vast majority of people would get results. Look at your own track record. The majority of people I work with come to me saying that they have been following a healthy diet fairly well for quite some time. This is all the evidence you need. If you have been following a healthy diet and did not get results then you need to accept, even though it is healthy in a general sense it does not work for you. Something needs to be changed or added to it.

If you change your mindset so you are following it in a ballpark of consistency then you should get results. The proof will be in the mirror and clothes size as well as how you feel. Some people reading this book will get some great results by just improving their mind set so that they can follow their current plan more efficiently. This is because they already have the right plan but simply need to follow it a little better. For the majority of people however they will most likely have to change both their mind set and their nutrition and exercise routines. For a smaller yet still significant proportion of people they will have to go much deeper and resolve blocking factors before they can get the results they want.

Finding the right plan

At the heart of the right plan is first developing the right mindset. Any plan that does not do this either requires your subconscious programming to be good enough to get results or requires will power. For the majority of people neither of these will be good enough to provide any long term results.

Once the mind is in place then you must identify the right foods for your body and then introduce exercise. This varies from person to person. It should incorporate the four areas of exercise; resistance, aerobic, core and flexibility training but the combination will vary depending on the person involved and their physiology.

Alongside this you should be looking for the underlying causal factors of why you are not in shape already. This can include looking at calorie intake, macronutrients, micronutrients, blood sugar, metal toxicity, spinal alignment, viruses, parasites, hormones and much more.

How far you have to take this search depends on how your body responds. For some people they could simply reduce wheat from three times a day to once a day to get results. For others they must eliminate dairy and other sensitive foods for many months while also undergoing a detoxification programme. Perhaps you just need to reduce calorie intake by 300 calories per day. How many things you will need to put in place and to what extent they need to be done depends on biochemical individuality and where you are in relation to your goals.

For some people getting results will be easy when they have the right mind set, while for others it is a much longer road. It is irrelevant how much of a journey awaits you compared to someone else because you will either do what it takes for results and look amazing or you will not. It does not matter if it is much harder or easier, the only thing that matters is the result.

When you discover the right plan and follow it you will see the body transform. You will have increased energy, body fat loss, reduction of food cravings, return to normal hunger patterns, improved fitness levels, more muscle tone, avoid illness, improvement of health issues, increased sex drive, higher body temperatures (increased resistance to the cold), clearer thinking patterns, better productivity and many more positive traits.

When it comes to finding the right plan you must have the right level and type of commitment as well as understanding knowledge means action. They represent the crux of success.

True commitment is doing the things that must be done, not the things you think should be done or would like to do. True commitment also includes committing to finding out the difference between these two things. Knowledge is what you do. It is not what is in your head or what you talk about but it is what you do.

When you really look at these terms you will see that they all are another way of saying action. This sums it all up. Action is the bridge between thoughts and reality, between dreaming about it and living it. It should become your only acceptable outcome or measure. For this is what solely determines your shape.

BEHAVIOUR CHANGE EXERCISES

Awareness –

Take a look at where you sit along the continuum of being in great shape. This will tell you how successful your plan has been so far unless you are a fake thin person.

Ask yourself what elements of your plan are out of place? Correlate your results to your actions to see how well the plan is working. For example, if you have been eating a low fat diet for 3 years and you are still the same weight then what does this suggest?

Questioning –

Why are you following this plan? What types of plan do people in great shape follow? How can you find out about what plan you should follow?

Intention –

Accept that your plan of action may be wrong or in need of refinement. Drop any pride or emotional attachment to it and instead focus solely on finding the solution to push things forwards. Touch your hand on your heart and say out loud Ten times:

"I seek out and follow the right plan to be successful"

Planning –

Check out the references at the back of the book and commit to reading some of these texts. Begin today the journey to finding the plan that works for you.

Emotional management –

A big block many people have is failing to believe that the general healthy advice could be so wrong. Evidence is the best way to change this emotion. Look at society, the evidence is clear to see. Most people are in awful shape let alone amazing shape. This suggests that the general advice must be wrong. The general population follow the general advice.

Whatever you believe is the process by which people get in shape, e.g. low carbs, low fat, lots of running etc look to the people who actually do this for their routine. How many get results and how many fail to progress? Almost every plan will fail many people while aiding others, e.g. overweight people on low carb or low fat diets, overweight marathon runners etc.

Remind yourself it is ok to have been wrong before about how to get in shape and give yourself permission to experiment with other plans and methodologies for getting into shape.

EXAMPLES OF THE TEN PRINCIPLES WITHIN YOUR PERSONALITY

You have now read about the ten principles of how people in amazing shape think differently to those who struggle to get results. It is important you understand the difference between knowing about these and living by them. From reading this book you are already aware of them but that does not mean you have them within your subconscious mind yet. The behaviour change programme in section four is designed to facilitate this process. Before we move onto this I want to help you understand the differences between "knowing" and "being" a little further. To do this I have outlined what it looks like when you have or have not got each of the principles within your personality.

Examples of Principle 1 – People in amazing shape know they deserve to achieve their goal and avoid making weight a covering issue.

When this is within your personality it becomes shown by the fact you do not accept second bests in the majority of situations. When you know it is your right to be in shape you just do what it takes to get results. I had one client who said to me in about my fitness goals, "do you not think it is selfish to focus on achieving your goals?" On the contrary, it is selfish to not achieve your goals. To help others you must always help yourself first. You must pull people up to your level. You are most effective at helping others when you have helped yourself first. When you have this attitude within your personality you will truly deserve to achieve your goal. You will feel worthy of success. This means you will avoid self sabotage and you are free to go on to achieve your goal.

When this characteristic is missing from your personality you will often find self sabotage brings you down. There will be an underlying general feeling of a lack of worthiness, you will feel that being in shape couldn't be for you. If your weight is a covering issue then you will be overcome with obsessions, fears and panics about all things to do with your body. When you do make progress with your body these will not lessen. You will think constantly about your goals yet not actually get that many behaviours done.

Examples of Principle 2 – People in amazing shape think looking good is important, inspirational and can be achieved alongside other goals in life

When you hold this attitude you get excited about the thought of achieving your goals. This spurs you into action.

You will often find yourself thinking how great it is to be in amazing shape. (As opposed to thinking how life would not be so bad if you were in shape).

When you have this attitude you will know how important your goals are and understand that there are also influences from other goals and demands in life. When these are conflicting you will pull something out of the bag and drop the excuses to gain at least parity in your behaviours until normal service can be resumed. You will understand that you can be in shape and be successful in other areas of your life.

If this element is missing you will regularly find other things get in the way of your exercise or nutrition. You will find your work, family, friends, hobbies etc always come before looking after your body. You will feel you have to achieve your goals as opposed to wanting to achieve them. Thoughts about your goals will also bring negative feelings as well.

Examples of Principle 3 – People in amazing shape commit to their goals through the power of action

When this is within your persona you find that you no longer spend hours telling people about what you are going to do but that you have already done it. This person measures their success by how many actions they have taken, end of story. They rarely use the words "I tried, I did my best, I have put a lot of effort in" because they are saying "I did this, I have done it, I am doing". It is all about action! They know that talk is cheap.

Until you have this attitude well and firmly developed you will find yourself justifying to anyone who will listen why you have not or could not have done something. Despite this you will still be out of shape.

When you have committed through action you will be free from resentment of having to do the tasks needed to bring success. You understand you need to do things to get into shape and look forward to the prospect. Those who do not have this aspect developed will be holding a lot of resentment at all things health and fitness.

Examples of Principle 4 – People in amazing shape use emotional outlets that do not involve food or drink

When you have developed emotional outlets other than using food and drink you will appear much calmer to your friends. They will ask why you never need to grab after food, why you are so disciplined. To you of course you will be naturally using more effective emotional strategies and thus these behaviours are just normal.

You will find you feel so much more fulfilled because of the effect you are having on your emotions instead of hiding from them under a mound of food. This will make you happier and you will radiate a different energy and glow to the world. This will bring better things into your life. With well developed coping strategies you are also more forgiving of yourself if you do use food during times of emotional stress. You will be able to create a good balance within your eating.

When this attitude is in place you will simply be happier as a person, look better and be more in control of your health and fitness than the average person. Without this attitude you will find that you always struggle to cut out your troublesome foods. You will find the success of your efforts is directly related to your emotional state. You will feel controlled by food and worry about it.

Examples of Principle 5 - People in amazing shape avoid making excuses

With this strongly developed within your personality you will rarely mention excuses in terms of your goals but rather mistakes, miscalculated strategies and learning experiences along the path to where you are now. You will not beat yourself up for the mistakes you have made but see them as minor setbacks when they happen which become invaluable learning experiences in the long term.

A weekend of binge eating may not be a bad thing if it revealed to you the emotional causes behind your eating patterns and therefore putting you on the pathway to success. When excuses are gone from your vocabulary everything is a learning experience. You will identify your excuses and try to overcome these problems while focusing on how to counterbalance any negative behaviours that are unavoidable.

Until you have developed this attitude you may find your life is one long sob story. Everything seems to get in the way and life is always against you. The story may sound tough but remember your body is not listening and you will be out of shape as a result from your lack of action.

Examples of Principle 6 - People in amazing shape take an interest in getting into shape and understand they are unique

When you have this in your personality you will find that you are reading articles, newsletters and books on the subjects surrounding your health. You will also feel totally bemused with how the entire, media, education system and world is so wrong with their advice. You just keep noticing day in day out that everyone is not even in a ball park of getting results in their health and fitness. You will look on in dismay at how most people are not even close to doing what their body needs for optimal functioning.

When this trait is missing you will be confused by the conflicting advice you hear and find it too much of an effort to try and sort through the facts. You will jump from one plan to another without much reasoning or logic and find yourself running around in a circle with little success.

Examples of Principle 7 – People in amazing shape are able to attain balance in life and have the best of both worlds

When you truly understand balance and achieving the best of both worlds you will be exactly where everyone who attempts a diet wants to be. You will be getting results yet still do not feel restricted or deprived. You will be enjoying all aspects of getting fit and feel relaxed about it all.

When you have attained balance in your life you will be relaxed around saying no to junk food yet also relaxed in having it occasionally. You will not need to play mind games with yourself.

Once you have mastered the ability to attain both from apparent either / or situations you will be loving life because you will have the best of both worlds. You will still have the social life you want yet also be able to achieve the results you desire. This will also feel like the natural behaviour pattern you want to do.

When this is missing from your personality you will find that you feel deprived throughout any attempt to get into shape. You will alternate between periods of being 'strict' and periods of 'letting it go'. The net result will be little progress if any. You will also find yourself continually making choices between either helping your body get in shape or choosing another option in life such as social functions or work etc. You will never get the balance right.

Examples of Principle 8 – People in amazing shape associate with others in amazing shape.

When you have the right compliment of friends you will be learning off everyone. You will learn by the mistakes of the people who are out of shape and by the success of those who are in shape. You will naturally find yourself joining groups which contain people in sensational shape. You will enjoy hanging out with like minded healthy and fit people.

When this is lacking you will find you do not know anyone who is in amazing shape. You will find other people continually drag you down and you hold various resentments and stereotypes about people in awesome shape.

Examples of Principle 9 – People in amazing shape incorporate their health and fitness attitudes into their personality

When you have the health and fitness traits needed for success within your personality you will be viewed as health conscious or a fitness freak by most people. It is not necessary to be a fitness freak to be successful but the average person's view of a fitness freak is probably someone who does exercise twice a week and even bothers to look at what they eat. With such a low bar I would be a little worried if the average person does not think you are a fitness freak / very health conscious.

When your health and fitness attitudes are within your personality you will have people asking you for advice. If this element is developed properly people will stop offering you junk food, under the assumption that you always say no. This does not mean you have to say no but not being harassed into it makes life a little easier.

When this trait is not developed, you will find yourself hiding your behaviours from other people. You will not want to make a fuss nor let people know how you act. People will not view you as health conscious and will continually offer or try to tempt you into negative health behaviours.

Examples of Principle 10 – Follow the right plan

This one is simple, you will be getting results. If not, then something is wrong. Either you are not sticking to the plan, the plan is wrong or the plan is fine but you have not gone in deep enough to resolve the underlying blocking factors. People in amazing shape find the plan that works for them and stick to it. Those in poor shape do not find the right plan and / or do not stick to it.

SECTION 4

HOW TO GET INTO AMAZING SHAPE

In the first section you learnt the basic principles that underlie the whole area of changing your mind and your body. In section two you discovered the major beliefs that prevent you from getting the body you want. Section three outlined the way people in amazing shape think and act differently to their out of shape counterparts.

This section focuses on how you can now go forwards to develop a breathtaking body both inside and out. To do this you need to:

1) Create a mindset so you can follow a nutrition and exercise regime that will produce results
2) Discover the right nutrition and exercise routine for you

3) Follow this plan and adjust to include blocking factors as is necessary to get the results you desire.
4) Enjoy being in amazing shape and inspire others to do the same.

This book has focused almost exclusively upon your mind set (stage 1) with very little "Eat this, avoid that" advice (stages 2 and 3). This is because the first stage of the process is about getting the mind prepared to follow a plan for the long term. It is more important to understand how your mind works and develop the thinking infrastructure for long term success than to find out what to eat tonight or tomorrow. When you have the mindset in place the rest will come to you naturally as a result of your behaviour patterns.

In this section I will show you how to create the mindset of someone in amazing shape. To do this you will need to focus your efforts upon creating a new style of thinking. This can be done by working on different areas of your mind set each day. I have also outlined a 15 week plan to help you go forwards to get results.

CREATING THE MINDSET OF SOMEONE IN AMAZING SHAPE

For long term success you will need to dedicate time to creating a mind set to achieve your goals. The 15 week plan in this chapter outlines what to do immediately upon finishing this book. For now understand simply that you will need to dedicate some time each day (even if just 5-10 minutes) to develop the right mind set for success. This is important because you have created your beliefs and behaviours over the last 10, 20 to 40 years plus. There is no way you can expect to reverse them all just by skimming through this book once. Continuous daily action is the only way to reverse such conditioning.

Even when you have developed the right mind set and are getting results you must still be wary of the daily bombardment you will come under. The success rate for long term body transformations is very low. You must continuously work on your mind in some form to keep ahead of the game.

YOUR DAILY BEHVAVIOUR CHANGE EXERCISES

Going forwards from today dedicate 10- 30 minutes each day to work on your mindset. Have this take priority over any exercise or gym routines or any other elements of your healthy living plan. Within your daily mind change time you can use any of the techniques listed below. Look to select one or more of these to use within your regime each day. Try to rotate the techniques listed below so that within a one to two weeks period you have covered each different one. Make sure you have joined my website newsletter for more articles, videos and much more to help you with your daily mind exercises – www.benwilsonuk.com

Reading / listening to this book

For optimal changes you need to not only read this book now, but ideally once a month for the next year. Yes! Once a month for the next year! You cannot receive this information too many times. With the amount of conditioning you have working against your efforts you simply need to be overloaded with an alternative point of view. Listening to an audio version of this book is also an effective way to drive the information into your subconscious.

Doing the behaviour change exercises from this book

The behaviour change exercises at the end of each of the ten principles are very effective at inducing behaviour change. You should ensure you do every exercise in the book however hard, boring or pointless you think they appear to be. The more you think about your behaviour, analyse and create solutions the sooner you will solve the problems that are preventing success.

Affirmations

The use of statements about how you want to act can be a powerful tool to implement behaviours into your mind. You would have seen an affirmation within each of the behaviour change exercises. Simply repeat each of these out loud to yourself. The more repetitions you do the better. Feel free to edit the words to fit your own circumstances or feelings. If you are familiar with the techniques of power affirmations or Psych-K then these can be even more effective. You need to bombard your mind with the beliefs you want to hold.

Anchors

You will recall in the blocking belief about food making you happy that there was an exercise to create an anchor for happiness. This was done by holding your thumb and first finger together on your left hand and spending two minutes thinking about a time where you felt really happy followed by two minutes thinking about a time you will be happy in the future.

You also saw how to create the anchor to induce the feelings of success that will come from achieving your goal. This was done by holding together your thumb and first finger on your right hand. Spend two minutes imagining the benefits of being successful in your health and fitness goals followed by two minutes of focusing on the behaviours that you must do to be successful.

The final anchor you have already created was for relaxation by holding your thumb and middle finger of your left hand together while spending two minutes thinking about a time you were very relaxed and followed by two minutes thinking about a time in the future you will be just as relaxed.

The more you practice creating these, the stronger the anchors will become and the easier it will be to use them for a quick emotional reminder while out and about in the real world. Simply hold the anchor together to induce happiness, relaxation or renewed motivation for your goal.

Permission

For any of the techniques discussed here to work you must make sure you have permission to be successful or your efforts will go unrewarded. Many people do not give themselves permission to achieve the results they want. They deny themselves the permission to feel happy, to be confident, to feel attractive or to put their emotional events and concerns behind them. A lack of permission is enough to prevent any of the strategies outlined so far from working. Linked to this is having an elaborate set of rules or difficult criteria to meet before you allow yourself to feel a certain way.

Perform the following exercise to give yourself permission to change and develop into the person you want to be. Continue until you feel it is ok to move forwards and achieve your goals. Return periodically to this exercise to ensure the feelings remain true to you. Say out loud and tap the EFT points (see www.benwilsonuk.com for tapping points).

"I give myself permission to feel happy exactly the way I am now, I give myself permission to achieve results, I give myself permission to move on emotionally, I give myself permission to release my fears, I give myself permission to change, I give myself permission to love myself exactly as I am today. I give myself permission to achieve my goals."

Value clarification

Your values are the collections of beliefs by which you aim to live your life. Sometimes there can be a conflict of values that are preventing your success. The greatest success and natural motivation comes when your health and fitness goals are aligned to your highest values. For example, if being a good parent is your highest value then you could view going to the gym as stealing time away from your children (therefore you rarely go) or that the gym makes you a better parent and serves your children by you being healthy (therefore you always go).

Sometimes people struggle to achieve their goals because they have a clash of values. For example, if being rich (value – money) is the most important thing to you and you hold an image of success which shows you being able to eat anything you want in a restaurant every night then there may be a clash of values. To feel "rich" (most important feeling to you) you will try to eat whatever you want in a restaurant. This may overpower and compromise the less important value of being in shape. While almost every person in amazing shape has looking good near the top of their value lists for most people this is not the case.

Therefore, if you can identify your highest values in life and link the benefits of doing the activities to get in shape as directly helping your highest values you will tap into an almost unlimited motivation resource, e.g. if religion or spirituality is your number one value you must link exercise and good nutrition as bringing you closer to God / making you more spiritual. If being a good mother is the most important thing to you then you must link how being in shape teaches your children to be healthy and how you save them worry by being so healthy.

This mental exercise is simply about spending time thinking, discussing or analysing your current values and then seeing how becoming successful in health and fitness develops these values further. Time spent reflecting on this is very powerful.

Learning emotional management strategies

You have seen throughout this book the relationship between emotions and success. To be able to control and manage your emotions is beyond crucial for success. To be able to do this you should first learn one or more of the various strategies available to you.

To handle emotions you can use one of the many different techniques discussed previously. This can include EFT, TFT, IEMT, CBT, NLP, Psych K etc. My favourite is EFT because it can be done easily on your own and is quick to learn. Follow the references in the back of the book to start your journey to mastering one or more of these techniques.

Many people try these techniques once or twice then quit saying they don't work. I can tell you this now, they all work to reduce emotions and can all be very powerful. However, you must dedicate time to learning how these processes work. You couldn't drive a car the first time you sat behind the wheel but that doesn't mean cars cannot get you from A to B. At the same time it doesn't mean these techniques are the grand saviour of everything but they are certainly helpful.

Ideally you will learn more than one strategy over time and to a fairly good standard. This will give you the skills to remove more than enough emotion to achieve your goals. Remember when discussing emotions, any positive changes have the potential to transform all areas of your life and not just your health and fitness goals. My website has plenty of information on these techniques and strategies.

Reducing emotions

Once you have become familiar with one of the techniques to reduce emotions, you must of course, apply it to your own stress! The fewer negative emotions you are experiencing, the easier it will be to eat the right foods and motivate yourself to exercise.

Reducing the emotional stress from past events -

Using your preferred emotional reduction strategy you should focus on specific events from the past that still evoke negative emotions today. We all have hundreds of these. The more you clear the negative emotions the weaker your desire to use addictive behaviours. In EFT circles this is called the personal peace procedure. It can take many months to reduce the numerous events within your mind-body. The unresolved events you hold may range from large to small issues, e.g. someone's death verses guilt because you broke the neighbour's window by accident. There are no rights or wrongs about what you should address, as any event removed will reduce your overall level of emotions experienced. For larger events it should be done with the help of a trained therapist.

Reducing current day emotional stress contributors

The way to address your present tense evaluations in life is two-fold, become content in the areas that are creating negative emotions and put in place a plan to move forward within these areas. The plan can be done using basic goal achievement, self help strategies and advice from people in the know. Contentment can be created by combining EFT with positive psychology principles. The exercise below identifies your current evaluations versus expectations in life. Use EFT on any areas you feel you are not living up to your expectations.

Life area	My evaluation now of where I am in this area	My expectation of where I wanted to be at this age	Expectation in 5 years
Love			
Family			
Friends			
Work			
Money			
Sex			
Recognition			
Spirituality			
Personality			
Health			
Body shape			
Hobbies			
Other:			

Contentment

Feeling content with yourself is a powerful way to reduce the emotions from events in your present tense. Accepting yourself, as you are, does not mean you will all of a sudden brainwash yourself into thinking you weigh 3 stone (42lbs / 19KG) less than what you actually weigh. It will however, free your mind up, ease pressure and allow you to see that you want to achieve your goals out of enjoyment and not because you 'have to' achieve them. This allows for faster progress and higher natural motivation.

To help you feel content perform EFT by tapping the various points until you feel more content about the situation. Use the structure as set out below:

Even though I haven't ____________ as I wanted to at my age, I deeply and completely accept myself for the way I am now".

e.g. "Even though I do not earn as much money as I wanted to at my age, I deeply and completely accept myself for the way I am now".

Present tense stresses

We all have stresses in our life that are immediate and must be addressed. These can easily knock you off track. Your day to day stresses are often directly related to your expectations. Your self-imposed expectations often cause the majority of the stress in any situation rather than the actual facts of the issue. For example, your expectation that all your work must be 100% correct, the kids must look perfect before school or that you must check all your emails each night, may create more problems than it solves. Take time to evaluate if any of your expectations are creating more harm than good.

You can also reduce stress by identifying what activities drain you and which energise you. Then look to reduce the former and increase the latter wherever possible.

Reducing the emotional stress from future worries

Using your preferred emotional reduction strategy look to identify the specific worries and concerns you hold about the future. These can range from smaller upcoming events to larger issues of life, death and spirituality.

Taking positive action is also a powerful way to reduce emotions from the future. This could be drawing up a plan of action, working towards a goal each day, studying about areas that are giving you concerns, e.g. reading books on spirituality, religion.

Developing ways to increase happiness

The more activities you do in your life that make you feel happy without using food or drink, the easier it will be to get results. You should look at increasing the activities that induce the different types of happiness. You will recall that there are four types of happiness; Enlightenment, Fulfilment, Satisfaction and Pleasure. These can be achieved by creating more love in your life (giving unconditionally over trying to receive), following your inspiration or by tuning into which activities bring satisfaction and pleasure. Deepening of your understanding around thought and happiness will also make it easier to access these feelings.

The more of these activities you do in your life, the happier you will be. Complete the table below by writing down as many activities as possible within each category. Then spend some time devising a way to actually do more of these in your life:\

Unconditional Love	Inspirational activities	Satisfying activities	Pleasurable activities

Spending time with people in amazing shape

When you spend time with likeminded individuals it charges your mind set to train harder, more intelligently and to focus on your nutrition. Spending time with people in shape discussing your health and fitness goals is a productive, enjoyable and necessary part of achieving high level performance. If you currently have no friends in great shape then spend time thinking where you could meet such people and get out there to meet them. You can also use websites such as You Tube to watch videos of people in amazing shape to see how they train, live etc. You can follow most celebrities you admire on Facebook or Twitter. You can join online groups (Facebook/NING etc) to connect with likeminded people.

You should also use this time to review your current relationships and interactions with people who are not in great shape. Look to develop plans of action so that you can reduce their negative influence upon you.

Studying techniques to get into shape

As discussed, stage 1 of your plan to get in amazing shape is to create the mind set needed for results. However, the sooner you learn stages 2 and 3 the faster the physical transformation will take place. Start learning about nutrition and exercise from sources at the back of this book, my websites, other websites, books, people and experts. Do not do this technique to the exclusion of the other mind and behaviour change techniques within this section. Use your time in this section to also plan out what you will do in the upcoming days in terms of nutrition and exercise etc.

Other strategies

I have detailed more than enough strategies for you to create substantial changes in your mind set and thus go on to achieving amazing results. The list above is by no means exhaustive, with many other strategies available to you including the many forms of meditation, hypnosis and other behaviour change techniques. The choice is varied but the results are the same. You become in control of your behaviours and emotions thus go on to achieve you goals.

YOUR 15 WEEK PLAN FOR SUCCESS

To help you start the process I have set out a 15 week plan below to get you going on your journey to being in amazing shape. If you are interested in going deeper with this then check out my behaviour change courses as listed in the further learning section.

Weeks 1 – 3 – Mind preparation phase

During this phase you are to focus solely on developing the right mindset. You are not to try any crazy diets, mad exercise routines or anything else to distract you from the main goal at hand which is developing the right mind set for future success.

Spend 30 minutes each day working on your mind set. Simply choose one of the many methods outlined previously. Each day look to either read this book, go through the behaviour change exercise at the end of each chapter, create an anchor, repeat affirmations, work on permission, think about your values, learn emotional reduction techniques, reduce emotions, work on increasing happiness, look for other people in great shape, handle people of negative influence or study techniques to get in shape.

For eating and exercise simply continue doing what you were or were not doing before. Ensure nothing takes priority over the 30 minutes of mind change activity you must do each day.

Weeks 4 – 6 – Follow your theory on how getting into shape works

One of the biggest blocks I have found, will be your very own beliefs of how weight loss works. Therefore it is often a good idea to try out your methodology to see if it actually works for you. After three weeks of mind training you should be able to follow most plans. Look to continue the mind exercises daily spending 10 – 30 minutes per day rotating through the various behaviour change techniques.

At the end of the week six review the progress you have or have not made. This should be measured along the lines of body fat, clothes size and sub clinical health issues, e.g. energy, sex drive, concentration, health problems. DO NOT use the weighing scales as your only measurement tool if at all. At the end of week 6, take some time to review progress. Broadly speaking you will either have:

1) Followed the plan and got good results – Plan is working!

2) Followed it but did not get results – Wrong plan and / or blocking factors.
3) Could not stick to it – Wrong plan / mind set issue. It is likely you are following a plan that is giving you nutritional cravings, making unrealistic demands etc and / or your mind set is not in the right place.

Weeks 7- 12 – Experimentation phase

After your week six review, if you got results, then you may continue with the plan and move into this stage only if you hit a plateau. If you did not get results or could not follow the plan, then start the experimentation phase as below. Throughout this phase continue the daily mind exercises for ideally 10- 30 minutes plus. The phase is designed to allow you to learn about how your body feel / reacts.

<u>Week 7 – Have no dairy or gluten grains.</u> Eliminate all dairy products and gluten grain based products. This means removing bread, cereals, pasta as well as obvious dairy products. Ensure you consume protein, carbohydrates and fat at each meal so you do not feel hungry. Experiment with the amounts of each to ensure hunger and cravings are removed. At the end of the week note down your feelings and changes in your body as you did after week six.

<u>Week 8 - Eliminate all fruits.</u> This week eat any food except fruit. Feel free to reintroduce dairy and gluten grains if you did not see major improvements during the previous

week. Ensure you consume protein, carbohydrates and fat at each meal so you do not feel hungry. At the end of the week note down your feelings and changes in your body.

Week 9 – Eat a high red meat diet – Look to increase the amount of red meat within your diet. Feel free to reintroduce foods if you did not see major improvements during the previous week. At the end of the week note down your feelings and changes in your body. Eat freely from any other food groups. Ensure you consume Protein, carbohydrates and fat at each meal so you do not feel hungry. At the end of the week note down your feelings and changes in your body

Week 10 – Eat no red meat – Eliminate all red meats from your diet. Feel free to eat freely from all any other food groups while allowing for information from previous experimental weeks. Ensure you consume protein, carbohydrates and fat at each meal so you do not feel hungry. At the end of the week note down your feelings and changes in your body

Week 11 – Stop cardio (if a regular exerciser) or start exercising (if you do no exercise) – Look to eat freely from any food group while allowing for information from previous experimental weeks. Ensure you consume protein, carbohydrates and fat at each meal so you do not feel hungry. If you are a regular exerciser stop all cardio and perform only weight training for your exercise routine. If you do not exercise then start doing some activity. Do not worry what type of exercise or feel you must join a gym. Just do anything to get your body moving. At the end of the week note down your feelings and changes in your body

Week 12 – Have water as your only drink – Eliminate all drinks and beverages apart from water within your diet. This includes tea, coffee, flavoured water, fruit juices, alcohol etc. Eat freely from any food groups. Ensure you consume protein, carbohydrates and fat at each meal so you do not feel hungry. At the end of the week note down your feelings and changes in your body

During this whole process be aware of detox reactions. These are negative symptoms that occur as a result of removing a sensitive food or substance. During these stages you can feel awful. If symptoms are severe then reintroduce the food group and look to reduce consumption over a longer period e.g. two week period before beginning the elimination week. This is especially important if you are cutting out caffeine related drinks. Do not battle through severe symptoms, simply extend the elimination week into a longer three week reduction phase. Be wary of removing too many foods so you are left with nothing left to eat. Use common sense in such situations.

Week 13 - 15 – Combine the best elements for rapid results

From the experimental weeks you should have begun to get an idea of what works well for you. Look to combine the best features into a plan and follow it for three weeks to see the effects on the body. Remember that one of the key attitudes of people in amazing shape is to see the information factually and not emotionally. If a favourite food, or a really so called "healthy" food makes you fat or feel bad, then do not ignore the information or try to justify it. Develop the mind until you see no longer want to eat it.

Week 15 plus

At this stage you have either:

1) Got some results –Continue the plan until you go onto to be in amazing shape. If you plateau at some point then see points 2 and 3 below.
2) Followed it but got no results – You need to try a more personalised plan and/or address blocking factors.
3) Did not really follow it – You need to develop your mind further against the backdrop of a sound plan of action tailored towards your mind-body.

Whichever option applies you have started your journey to achieving the body you want. You must now continue with it.

FINAL WORDS

Thank you for reading this far and I wish you the greatest success in the future. Remember you are an amazing person and you can achieve all your goals. Simply be honest and open with yourself about where you are weakest and then study this area. Persistence will pay off and results will come. Go forwards from today and start changing your mind set so that you are on auto pilot to create an amazing body transformation that will not only benefit you but also inspire others to change. Keep in contact with me in one the many ways available on the internet today.

Ben Wilson

FURTHER LEARNING

To join my weekly newsletter and to view the referenced videos, behaviour change courses please visit:

www.benwilsonuk.com

Emotional Freedom technique (EFT):
http://www.emofree.com

Thought Field Therapy (TFT):
http://www.rogercallahan.com

Psych-K:
http://www.psych-k.com

Cognitive Behaviour Therapy (CBT):
http://www.nacbt.org

Neuro-linguistic Programming (NLP):
http://www.richardbandler.com
http://www.johngrinder.com

Integral Eye Movement Therapy (IEMT)
http://www.integraleyemovementtherapy.com

Good Websites –

www.geniuscatalyst.com – Self-help, Three Principles &Happiness
www.threeprinciplesmovies.com – Three Principles website.
www.mercola.com – Largest Natural Health website.

Books about positive psychology and creating happiness:

Feel Happy Now – Michael Neill
Positive Psychology – Charlotte Style

Books on Nutrition / Exercise to open your mind to get results:

How To Eat, Move and Be Healthy – Paul Chek
The Fat Loss Bible – Anthony Colpo
The Metabolic Typing Diet – William Wolcott
$29 Billion Reasons To Lie About Cholesterol – Justin Smith
The Mood Cure - Julia Ross
Nourishing Traditions – Sally Fallon

REFERENCES

1 – Biochemical Individuality - Dr Roger Williams (Keats 1998)

2 – William Wollcott – Health Excel System of Metabolic Typing – www.healthexcel.com

3 – Self made Chick - One Word that Can Change Your Reality and Perception of What Is Possible – (http://selfmadechick.com/)

http://selfmadechick.com/2007/09/28/one-word-that-can-change-your-reality-and-really-piss-off-other-people/

4 – There are numerous possible references including -

The National Diet and Nutrition Survey: adults aged 19 to 64 years L Henderson, J Gregory, G Swann (Office of National Statistics, UK)

http://tna.europarchive.org/20110116113217/http://www.food.gov.uk/science/dietarysurveys/ndnsdocuments/ndnspreviousssurveyreports/

Dietary fat is not a major determinant of body fat – Willet WC, Leibel RL (Am J Med 2002) http://www.ncbi.nlm.nih.gov/pubmed/12566139

5 – Predictably Irrational: The Hidden Forces that Shape Our Decisions Dan Ariely – Harper Collins (2009)

6 – United Nations – World Population Prospects 2006 Revision (www.un.org)

7 – World Health Organisation – Tobacco Atlas (http://www.who.int/tobacco/statistics/tobacco_atlas/en/)

8 – Nutrition and physical Degradation – Weston A. Price (Keats 1997)

See also the Price Pottenger Foundation – http://www.ppnf.org/

AUTHOR BIOGRAPHY

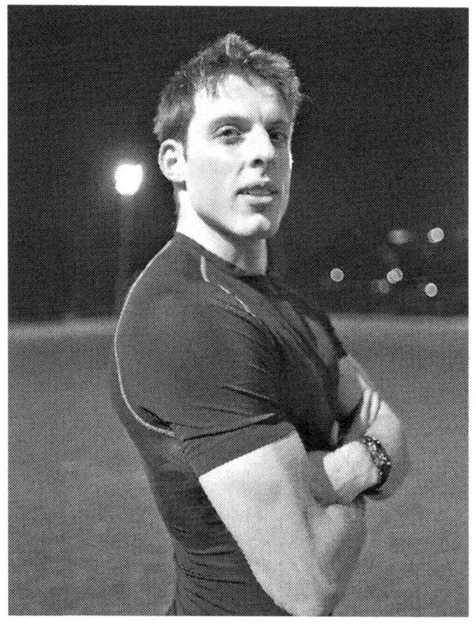

Ben Wilson

Ben is a personal trainer, nutritionist and behavioural change coach. He has been helping people lose weight and get into shape for over 10 years. He has worked with almost every possible type of client from professional athletes to post heart attack patients, business executives and stay at home mums. He has gained a unique insight into the field of body transformations through meeting thousands of people trying to get into shape covering all types of body shape from jaw dropping six packs to 20 stone (127kg) teenagers. Ben has discussed health and body transformations with people from all over the globe having visited over 50 countries and visiting gyms throughout the world ranging from a karaoke singing gym in Cambodia to state of the art facilities in California.

Ben has studied various behaviour change and emotional management strategies. These include Emotional Freedom Technique (EFT), Psych-K and spiritual healing. He has combined this knowledge with techniques used in Neuro-linguistic programming (NLP) and Cognitive Behaviour Therapy (CBT) and the research of people in shape versus those out of shape. He has also studied the 'Three Principles' and their application to stress and happiness.

In addition to this he possesses a degree in Chemistry from the University of Cardiff and has continued his study through looking at the fields of personalised nutrition, Metabolic Typing and Functional Diagnostic Nutrition. A qualified personal trainer his studies in strength and conditioning led him to write the book 'Rugby Fitness Training: A Twelve Month Conditioning Programme'.

A regular in the media Ben has made numerous TV and Radio appearances and often appears in the printed press. Ben runs a very popular weekly newsletter containing videos articles and information about changing your mind and body.

Made in the USA
Middletown, DE
11 September 2021